LIFE'S DELICATE BALANCE

LIFE'S DELICATE BALANCE

GUIDE TO CAUSES AND PREVENTION OF BREAST CANCER

CHEMICAL CARCINOGENS

IONIZATION RADIATION

ENDOCRINE DISRUPTERS — BREAST CANCER

GENETIC INTERACTIONS

Janette D. Sherman, M.D.

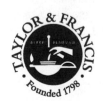

USA	Publishing Office	Taylor & Francis 29 West 35th Street New York, NY 10001-2299 Tel: (212)216-7800
	Distribution Center	Taylor & Francis 47 Runway Road, Suite G Levittown, PA 19057-4700 Tel: (215)269-0400 Fax: (215)269-0363
UK		Taylor & Francis 11 New Fetter Lane London EC4P 4EE Tel: 011 44 207 583 9855 Fax: 011 44 207 842 2298

LIFE'S DELICATE BALANCE

1 2 3 4 5 6 7 8 9 0

A CIP catalog record for this book is available from the British Library.

Library of Congress Cataloging-in-Publication Data

Sherman, Janette D.
Life's delicate balance : a guide to causes and prevention of breast cancer / Janette D. Sherman.
    p.   cm
Includes bibliographical references and index.
ISBN 1-56032-869-X (alk. paper). — ISBN 1-56032-870-3 (alk. paper)
1. Breast — Cancer Popular works. I. Title.
TD883.17 .H36   1999
363.739'2—dc2l

99-35846
CIP

CONTENTS

ACKNOWLEDGMENTS

There are many people to whom I am indebted for help in getting this book into print. Without their suggestions, criticism, and support, it would have been an even more difficult task. I have carefully considered each offering of information and criticism, and have tried to incorporate the many ideas and points of view into the book. I give thanks to all who have contributed to this effort, named and not named.

I give thanks to author and poet, Dr. Sandra Steingraber; to Dr. Lewis Walker, Chairman of the Department of Sociology at Western Michigan University, for reading the entire manuscript; and to Janet Collins, the prime organizer of the First World Conference on Breast Cancer; each of whom read the entire manuscript and provided valuable suggestions. I thank Marcia Marks, environmental activist, who read much of the manuscript and posed questions needing to be addressed.

I thank Dr. Ernest Sternglass, Dr. Jay Gould, Dr. Rosalie Bertell, and Dr. John Gofman, who gave of their time, provided fascinating and valuable information and suggestions, and critiqued portions of the radiation chapters.

I thank Dr. Michael Anbar for background material on thermography and for his critique of the chapter on mammography.

I appreciate the receipt of background materials, suggestions, and critique of individual chapters provided by Judy Brady, Helena Baldyga, Eve Clute, Janet Collins, Jane Gould, Karen McDonell, Hope Nemiroff, Dorothy Golden Rosenberg, Leonard Schroeter, Rose Marie Williams, Dr. Ruth Allen, Dr. Myron Mehlman, and Dr. Jay Nuckols, and encouragement from Dr. Jack Mongar.

I thank Judy Ochs, spirited, bright, and talented breast cancer thriver who provided the illuminating interviews that are included herein.

I give thanks to the dedicated environmental activists on Long Island, and especially to Mary Dowden, Elsa Ford, Miriam Goodman, and Mary Joan

Shea. I thank the activists from the Washington Toxics Coalition, the Rachel Carson Council, the First World Conference on Breast Cancer, and the brave and committed women I have met from the Virginia and Pennsylvania Breast Cancer Coalitions.

Lastly, my heartfelt thanks goes to my husband, Donald Nevinger, whose Smithsonian and internet research turned up fascinating background information, who read endless revisions, organized stacks of research materials, and was totally supportive when I had too many hours at the computer. I appreciate his thoughtfulness, encouragement, and support that has never wavered.

INTRODUCTION

We shall require a substantially new manner of thinking
if [human]kind is to survive.
—Albert Einstein

Twenty years ago, while serving on an advisory committee to the U.S. Environmental Protection Agency for the Toxic Substances Control Act, I was asked to write a short article on the issue of risks and benefits from exposure to chemicals. I called the paper "Cancer—Our Social Disease."[1] It seemed then, and it is clear now, that winning the so-called war on cancer will not be accomplished by physicians, scientists, pharmaceutical corporations, epidemiologists, geneticists, nor by the thousands employed in various governmental agencies and universities at home and abroad. It will be won by people who understand the connection between the loss of personal health and worldwide pollution from toxic chemicals, ionizing radiation, and endocrine-altering chemicals.

Anyone who doubts that prevention of cancer lies not in the realm of politics and economics need only read recent medical commentary attacking scientists who publish data linking chemicals and radiation to cancer. "Chemophobia, the unreasonable fear of chemicals, is a common public reaction to scientific and media reports suggesting that exposure to various environmental contaminants pose a threat to health,"[2] wrote a researcher whose work is supported generously by chemical and pharmaceutical corporations. Appearing a month later in the same journal that carried the above quote was a review of Dr. Sandra Steingraber's book, Living Downstream. It said "the work product of an environmentalist is controversy," and added that the book "frightens, at times misinforms, and then scorns genuine efforts at cancer prevention through lifestyle change."[3] The writer of this critique is the Director of Medicine and Toxicology for W. R. Grace & Company, which paid $8 million to settle claims brought by the families of seven Woburn, Massachusetts, children and an adult who developed leukemia after consuming water shown to be contaminated by chemicals dumped by that company. Now that the events of the Woburn contamination have been documented in the book A Civil Action[4] and in the movie by the same name, perhaps the public will begin to understand the undercurrents propelling the cancer epidemic, and blocking its reversal.

The tactic of labeling as controversial factors that adversely affect health and the environment is a common ploy used to control the message. "Controversy" is invoked to shut out discussion and alternative points of view. As long as the purveyors of toxic exposures can persuade the public to believe that there is reason not to consider a point of view, nothing will be done to change the current unacceptable reality of the cancer epidemic.

Some scientists and lay persons will not agree with my analysis of the links between chemicals, radiation, and endocrine disrupters and cancer. Many will demand more "proof," cite research that failed to demonstrate clear connections between "substance-X" and cancer, or suggest the need for more research. I encourage honest skepticism in the search for scientific verity, and encourage research, that is, independent research, free from economic pressures. However, while we do yet one more study, the Precautionary Principle must take precedence. This means we must take action to safeguard the health of the public and of the environment in the face of uncertainty.

I challenge the reader: If cancers are not caused by chemicals, endocrine-disrupting chemicals, and ionizing radiation, what are the causes? How else can one explain the doubling, since 1940, of a woman's likelihood of developing breast cancer, increasing in tandem with prostate and childhood cancers? Parallel with cancer has been the increase in chemical and nuclear industries. Do that many women have faulty "lifestyles"? Did the children in Woburn develop leukemia because of their faulty "lifestyle"? Or did they get sick because they drank water contaminated with chlorinated solvents?

While the diagnosis and treatment of cancer properly falls within the medical profession, all too often, physicians have failed to ask the pertinent questions as to why a patient developed cancer. Why do so few physicians probe into the environmental, workplace, and lifestyle history of their patients? Is it lack of training? Not enough time? Lack of curiosity? Given the current state of medicine and science, the prevention of cancer is clearly in the realm of economics and politics, and the ramifications have profound social consequences.

I am a physician, and my perspective on cancer and its many causes developed while listening to and examining some 8000 patients for the past 30-

plus years. My growing frustration over the lack of knowledge about causal links to disease by patients and their physicians, the lack of questioning as to causes of illness, and even worse, the lack of curiosity as to why a person got sick, led me to write Chemical Exposure and Disease, now in its second edition. The new book you are reading now, Life's Delicate Balance: Causes and Prevention of Breast Cancer, continues as an extension of my previous book.

As much as entrenched economic powers fear loss of profit, the other side of the economic equation—the human and economic costs of cancer—must be addressed. Staggering are the economic costs for hospital stays, medical examinations, laboratory tests, pharmaceuticals, special equipment, yes, even funeral services, and on and on. The destruction of so much of our earth's resources—water, air, soil, forests, food—is intricately linked to the worldwide cancer epidemic.

No less are the costs of pain inflicted on the patient, the patient's spouse, family, friends, coworkers, and society at large. The talent, skills, and productivity lost by persons suffering from cancer, undergoing surgery, radiation, chemotherapy, and recuperation are irreplaceable. "The average woman killed by breast cancer loses 20 years off her life. Thus, with approximately 46,000 women killed each year by breast cancer, we are now losing nearly a million person-years of experienced, productive women from this disease."[5] For those women, suffering alone, the physical and emotional burdens of cancer are rarely considered or mentioned. These all are part of an increasingly large economic and social burden.

My interest in social disruption as a consequence of cancer was expanded when, in 1993, I was appointed both an Adjunct Professor of Sociology and an Associate Member in the Graduate Faculty at Western Michigan University. It is in this larger context where the burdens of cancer upon the person, the family, and society are played out. This social, economic, and political arena is where we must focus and act if we are to achieve prevention of cancer. Defeating cancer requires understanding causes, and then addressing the factors in those causes: scientific, medical, political, economic, and social.

While not exhaustive, this book is intended to be a source of information about known links to cancer, "lifestyle" included. May this information provide a framework to expand this knowledge. This book is dedicated to all who are willing to work for prevention.

JANETTE D. SHERMAN

REFERENCES

1. Sherman, J. D. Cancer—Our social disease. CBE Environmental Review. pp. 7–9, 1978.
2. Safe, S. H. Xenoestrogens and breast cancer. New Engl. J. Med. 337(18): 1303–1304, 1997.
3. Berke, J. H. Book Reviews, Living Downstream: An Ecologist Looks at Cancer and the Environment. New Engl. J. Med. 337(21): 1562, 1997.
4. Harr, Jonathan. A Civil Action, Random House, New York. 498 pages, 1995.
5. Montague, P. Rachel's Environment & Health Weekly. #571. November 6, 1997.

1

ALL LIFE IS CONNECTED
CANCER IN HUMANS AND WILDLIFE

Man has lost the ability to foresee and to forestall.
He will end by destroying the earth.
—Albert Schweitzer, quoted in *Silent Spring*

WILDLIFE-HUMAN LINKS

It may be that biologists, rather than physicians, will be the major contributors to the health of our planet and its people. It was Rachel Carson, a biologist, who researched and wrote of the harm to wildlife caused by the combined action of pesticides and radiation. In the tradition of the observant biologist is Theo Colborn, who, with her colleagues, provided a significant breakthrough in understanding the hormonal effects of environmental contaminants. In July 1991, a gathering of some of the world's most astute scientists was held at the Wingspread Conference Center in Wisconsin[1] where they defined the pattern of diverse endocrine malfunction seen throughout the animal kingdom. They revealed a picture of the *Brave New World* we should rigorously seek not to leave as a legacy to our children.

The conferees, studying wildlife over the globe, described ominous findings of disease and death linked to environmental pollution. Exposure to toxic chemicals that possess unintended hormonal actions has resulted in anatomic, physiologic, reproductive, carcinogenic, and behavioral abnormalities across all forms of animal life: in mollusks, fish, birds, seals, and rodents. These creatures are to we humans as canaries were to the miners. We must understand that the destruction of eons of evolutionary function and development in wildlife foreshadows destruction of the entire biosphere, humans included.

1

These widespread adverse effects were attributed to xenoestrogens. *Xeno-* comes from a Greek origin, meaning "foreign." Foreign itself is not bad: else how do we share and spread culture and ideas? But xenoestrogens are less foreigners than invaders, gaining entrance by the Trojan horse of seemingly harmless routes: milk, meat, cheese, fish, the products we use to nourish ourselves and families. Like the invaders of Troy, after the xenoestrogens gain entrance to the bodies of animals and humans alike, they weaken defenses and wreak their harm of cancer, hormonal disruption, immunological abnormalities, and birth defects.

Xenoestrogens are an insidious enemy, but they have had help from powerful allies: the purveyors of products and chemicals, and legislators, regulators, and scientists reluctant to bite the money-laden hands that feed them.

Wingspread researchers found that birds exposed to xenoestrogens show reproductive failure, growth retardation, life-threatening deformities, and alterations in their brains and liver function.[2] "There is direct experimental evidence for permanent [organizational] effects of gonadal steroids on the brain as well as reproductive organs *throughout life*."[3] This means that off-spring whose brains have been altered are unable to function as had their parents. They become different in ability or function.

This means that the sea of hormonally active chemicals in which the fetus develops may change forever the health and function of the adult, and in some cases, may alter the course of an entire species.[4] Worldwide there are reports of declining sperm counts[5] and reduced ratio in births of male babies.[6] Without the capacity to reproduce, a species ceases to exist. Extinction is forever; a species loss has never been reversed.

The data derived from animal observations are unequivocal: breast and genital cancers, genital abnormalities, interference with sexual development, and changes in reproductive behavior are all expressions of a root cause. A possible connection between women with breast cancer and those having children with reversed sexual orientation is a question that bears study. This is not an idea from science fiction, considering what we have learned from observing wildlife and the effects of inappropriate hormonal influence upon the breast, brain, and reproductive organs. If an unequivocal answer were to emerge from human observation, it could have a significant impact upon the prevailing political and economic landscape, and may finally settle the nature or nurture issue of sexual orientation.

SILENT SPRING—SILENT WOMEN

Considering the accumulated knowledge linking chemical and radioactive contamination of the environment with increasing breast cancer rates means we must focus our energies and efforts on prevention.

Early were the eloquent words and pleas for prevention from Rachel Carson. Her book, *Silent Spring*, originally published in 1962, while she herself was suffering from breast cancer, is still a bestseller. Ms. Carson documented wholesale killing of species; animals, birds, fish, insects; the destruction of food and shelter for wild creatures; failure of reproduction; damage to the nervous system; tumors in wild animals; increasing rates of leukemia in children; and chronicled the pesticides and chemicals known at that time to cause cancer. This was over *30 years ago!*

Carson's is a book for every citizen, for without understanding of our collective actions and permissions, we cannot govern democratically. In Australia, a citizen is required to vote. In the United States, proclaimed by some politicians as the "greatest democracy on earth," often fewer than 50% bother to vote in a major election. Of those who do take the time to register and vote, few are sufficiently alert and/or educated to vote with intelligence, thought, and compassion. Requiring participation in the governance of ones' own country is not a bad idea. Requiring thoughtful voting may be more difficult, especially when it comes to such issues as cancer, pesticide use, consumer products, nuclear radiation, toxic chemicals, and environmental destruction. Taking this thought one step further, this democracy could do far worse than to require reading of *Silent Spring* as a requirement to vote! Radical? Perhaps. But is the ongoing cancer epidemic any less radical?

One successor to Ms. Carson has emerged in the person of Sandra Steingraber, an ecologist, poet, and scientist. In her book, *Living Downstream,* she writes eloquently of the connections between environmental contamination and cancer. Dr. Steingraber was diagnosed with bladder cancer at age 20, a highly unusual diagnosis in a woman, a young woman, a nonsmoker and nondrinker. She pursued the question, why? She realized a connection with our wild relations and she asks:

> Tell me, does the St. Lawrence beluga drink too much alcohol and does the St. Lawrence beluga smoke too much and does the St. Lawrence beluga have a bad diet ... is that why the beluga whales are ill? ... Do

you think you are somehow immune and that it is only the beluga whale that is being affected?[7]

The portion of Dr. Steingraber's book that struck me most personally was when she says:

> First, even if cancer never comes back, one's life is utterly changed. Second, in all the years I have been under medical scrutiny, no one has ever asked me about the environmental conditions where I grew up, even though bladder cancer in young women is highly unusual. I was once asked if I had ever worked with dyes or had been employed in the rubber industry. (No and no.) Other than these two questions, no doctor, nurse, or technician has ever shown interest in probing the possible causes of my disease—even when I have introduced the topic. From my conversations with other cancer patients, I gather that such lack of curiosity in the medical community is usual.[8]

I take her words as an indictment of the medical and scientific establishment, whose point of view must be changed. Certainly the lack of curiosity among physicians, scientists, policymakers, and politicians has contributed to the epidemic of illness among humans and wildlife alike.

An equally talented woman is Terry Tempest Williams, an ecologist and wildlife researcher, whose book, *Refuge: An Unnatural History of Family and Place,* tells the story of her Utah family, whom she labels "a clan of one-breasted women." Ms. Williams contrasts the life-affirming awareness of the Great Salt Lake wildlife refuge against the erosion-of-being, as cancer takes away the women in her family: her mother, her grandmothers, and six aunts. She writes: "I cannot prove that my mother Diane Dixon Tempest, or my grandmothers, Lettie Romney Dixon and Kathryn Blackett Tempest, along with my aunts, developed cancer from nuclear fallout in Utah. But I can't prove that they didn't."[9]

Times are changing. It is becoming impossible to ignore the carnage of endocrine-disrupting chemicals, nuclear radiation, and chemical carcinogens, alone and in combination, invading nearly every family with cancer.

Facing this reality may be too much for some people, afraid to look, or afraid of being the next victim. The story of cancer is not an easy one, and neither is cancer. But if we do not exert our efforts to prevent this disease, we doom our children and grandchildren to repeat our collective errors.

What does it take to change from environmental destruction and random killing to affirmation of life? Can the protection of life for ourselves and our environment be accomplished by women with breast cancer; the women at risk for breast cancer; the families of breast cancer victims? Who should lead? If we citizens can't and don't try, what are our alternatives?

REFERENCES

1. Colburn, T., Clement, C., Eds. Chemically-Induced Alterations in Sexual and Functional Development: The Wildlife/Human Connection. Princeton Scientific Publishing Co., Inc. Princeton, NJ. 403 pages. 1992.

2. Fox, G. A. Epidemiological and pathobiological evidence of contaminant-induced alterations in sexual development in free-living wildlife. pp. 147–158. In: Colburn, T., Clement, C., Eds. Op. cit.

3. vom Saal, F. S., Montano, M. M., Wang, M. H. In: Colburn, T. Clement, C., Eds. Op. cit., pp. 17–83.

4. Lutz, D. No conception. The Sciences. 36(1): 12–15, 1996.

5. Swan, S., Elkin, E. P., Fenster, L. Have sperm densities declined? A reanalysis of global trend data. Environ. Health Perspect. 105(11): 1228–1232, 1997.

6. Davis, D. L., Gottlieb, M. B., Stampnitzky, J. R. Reduced ratio of male to female births in several industrial countries. J. Amer. Med. Assoc. 279(13): 1018–1023, 1998.

7. Steingraber, S. Living Downstream. Addison Wesley, Reading, MA. p. 139, 1997.

8. Ibid., pp. 137 and 138.

9. Williams, Terry Tempest. Refuge: An Unnatural History of Family and Place. Vintage Books, Division of Random House, New York. p. 286. 1991.

2

The Delicate Balance of Life

How Cancer Grows

That life will never come again
Is what makes life so sweet.
—Emily Dickinson, poem no. 1741

Perhaps the number one scientific topic for the last decade of this century has been the identification of genetic links to disease. But it is well to remember that genetic means more than merely inherited. We know that most babies arrive on this earth with fully functioning genetic systems, despite varying ethnic backgrounds. While some cancers may arise from an inherited genetic defect, we know that many more arise from damage to the genetic machinery of *normal* body cells, damage that occurs during a lifetime. Genetic damage is the result of exposure to certain chemicals and/or various forms of radiation, and the damage occurs *randomly*. Genetic damage can also result from the formation of free radicals during normal metabolic processes. It is important to understand that cancer develops in *healthy* people . . . previously healthy people. We develop cancer when our bodies, normally functioning, are altered by submicroscopic forces, chemical and physical.

First let's look at normal cell growth. Life is chemistry in action, the switching on and off of life-giving systems and genes. All life is subject to the rules of chemistry, from the smallest virus to the largest animals, humans included.

All human life begins as two single cells, an egg and a sperm, that combine into one and develop into the miracle of a new being. An infant, a bird, even some plants begin this way. Two cells double to become 4, which double again and again to 16, 32, 64, on and on. But the developing being doesn't form randomly. The nervous system, the limbs, the heart, each develops in its own time, place, and form, directed by chemical messages embedded in each cell's genetic material.

The sequence of switches, the timing, the combinations, the number, the chemical milieu are all critical, else the developing being fails to thrive or is born with physical or developmental defects. We have learned that the cells of the newborn may already hold the key to the destruction of the future adult.

Each of us, inside our covering of skin, is composed of organs, made of various tissues, composed of cells. Our cells, in turn, are complex factories of life-sustaining biological processes, under control of genes that are composed of deoxyribonucleic acid (DNA). Our existence results from an expression of DNA components, complex in number and arrangement. We humans have 46 chromosomes in the nucleus of each cell. Inside of each chromosome are from 50,000 to 100,000 genes, made of DNA, the carriers of the genetic code—our personal and unique biological, physiological, and human history. That's 2.3 million to 4.6 million separate entities *for each cell,* developed over millennia, and programmed to work in time-dependent and environment-dependent coordination. Damage to any one of these separate entities may cause a cell to go awry. The life of every plant and animal is derived from similar genetic components.

Each cell in a person's body contains genes identical to every other cell. Whether a cell develops and functions as a liver cell or a thyroid cell depends upon which genes are "switched on" or "switched off" in which sequence, in which combination, and at which particular time.

Switching-off, or suppression of cell activity, is a necessary event that happens in adult and embryo cells alike. A human needs two eyes of just the right size and in the right place, one nervous system, complete and functioning, and a heart, with all chambers intact and in the right place. We cannot live with organs of uncontrolled size, nor with organs that do not properly function.

The DNA itself consists of a sequence of just four simple chemicals. These can be arranged and rearranged in different order and patterns to make different genes. Differences in arrangement make possible personal differences, even between members of the same family.

These chemicals of life are named adenine (A), thymine (T), cytosine (C), and guanine (G). These are relatively simple chemicals: adenine and guanine are purines, and cytosine and thymine are pyrimidines. A is always paired with T, and G with C. When each is attached to a simple sugar it forms the basic stuff of DNA. The arrangement and sequence of the purines and pyrimidines are like notes on pages of music. Their arrangement and sequence determine whether a song, or whether cacophony and static results. The conductor of this symphony of life is DNA, the double helix on which the notes are arranged. It is this song, this entire symphony, that transmits messages to the organism to produce proteins, enzymes, hormones, the energy systems—all the processes that make up life.

DNA carries the genetic code of all living entities—plant and animal alike. It is DNA that determines the uniqueness of each person. It is DNA that is passed to the offspring from the parents. It is DNA that controls all life-giving processes; thus to understand cancer, we must understand life and its processes. Life is both hardy and delicate at the same time. Damage to the genetic machinery of individual cells can trigger a series of miscalculations, altering a cell's normal function. When a gene is damaged by radiation or chemicals, or receives misinformation from a chemical messenger, and the mistaken signal is not corrected, the result is inappropriate or uncontrolled growth. This is the basis of cancer.

Figure 2.1
Steps in the cancer process.

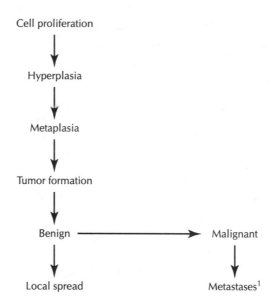

Cell proliferation

Hyperplasia

Metaplasia

Tumor formation

Benign ⟶ Malignant

Local spread   Metastases[1]

Cancer develops in *healthy* people. Cancer strikes children and adults alike. Cancer is *life uncontrolled* and occurs when a chemical cascade is set in motion that is difficult-to-impossible to reverse.

Following various steps along the way, from normal to frankly abnormal cells, provides understanding of the cancer process. See Figure 2.1. Cells can be studied under the microscope and tested with biological techniques. These studies show that neoplasia, literally "new growth," proceeds in a sequential fashion. That is, increase in the number of cells (proliferation); increase in size of each cell (hyperplasia); change in the basic structure (metaplasia); to frank tumor growth. Tumors may be either benign or malignant (cancerous), and each can spread locally and/or to distant sites.

These same uncontrolled processes occur throughout the living world: in humans, fish, turtles, birds, cattle, cats, dogs, even plants. All living creatures can develop the uncontrolled growth we call cancer. No life is exempt from cancer. Claims have been made that sharks don't develop cancer, but alas, they too succumb to cancer. To learn more about this, I visited the laboratory of Dr. John Harshbarger, Director of the Tumor Registry in Lower Animals for the Smithsonian and now at George Washington University. Dr. Harshbarger showed me tumors taken from sharks, benign and malignant, and from various organs. He explained that cancer development in these animals was a function of where the sharks had lived, in clean or polluted waters.

Alteration of the kind, sequence, or arrangement of DNA's components can change irreversibly the function and growth of a person, animal, or plant. Alterations in reproductive cells, the sperm or the egg, may be transmitted to the offspring, changing the life of that offspring, expressed as functional or physical defects, and with the potential to be transmitted to future generations. Defects in an offspring result from damage to the germ cells or to the embryo/fetus as it is developing.

Alterations in any of the other cells of the body, called somatic cells, may result in cancer. Cancer, the body's somatic cells gone awry, can be considered the destructive offspring of the body's tissues. A variety of insults, chemical and radiant energy, can change the function or form of an *originally normal* cell, sending it on the path to malignancy.

Changes can occur in any of the steps of normal cellular function: simple repair, chromosomal expression, gene alterations or deletions, enzyme changes, and amino acid substitutions. We have learned that even irritation, as from chronic formaldehyde exposure, results in increased cell-turnover, the need for repair, and the potential for interference with repair. This cascade helps explain not only hyperplasia, but the progression to metaplasia and cancer.[2,3] Some alterations may be reversed by a cell's innate repair mechanisms; some alterations may go unnoticed; but other alterations become permanent and life-threatening, as when a cancer begins.

Like reproductive development, cancer starts with a single cell and by doubling and doubling, grows until a mass may be felt, as a lump in one's breast. Left unchecked, the growth may invade neighboring tissues. Sometimes cells break off and travel by the blood and lymph to local and distant parts of the body. These distant growths are called metastases.

Progressing through this book, the reader will find information concerning agents that alter the way cells grow and function. Included in the discussion are descriptions of specific agents. These agents include hormones, pesticides, industrial chemicals, and nuclear radiation. Included are some sources of these damaging agents, and steps we can take to stop the ongoing assault on life called cancer.

REFERENCES

1. Sherman, J. D. Chemical Exposure and Disease. Princeton Scientific Publishing Co., Inc. Princeton, NJ, p. 213, 1994.
2. Graftstrom, R. C., Fornace, A. J. Jr., Autrup, H., Lechner, J. F., Harris, C. Formaldehyde damage to DNA and inhibition of DNA repair in human bronchial cells. Science. 220(4593): 216–218, 1983.
3. Sherman, J. D. Op. cit., pp. 109–111.

3

RISKS FOR BREAST CANCER
WE ALL ARE AT RISK

When you go out into the world, watch out for traffic,
hold hands and stick together.
—Robert Fulghum[1]

The popular and scientific press each make much of a woman's risk for developing breast cancer. What do these risks imply and are they really risks? Traditionally mentioned risks, including "lifestyle" factors, are implicated in perhaps 30% of breast cancers. The risks are listed below, in no particular order. These include:

A. History of breast cancer in mother or sister
B. Early onset of menarche
C. Late onset of menopause
D. Never pregnant, or first full-term pregnancy after age 30
E. Not breast feeding an infant
F. Obesity and/or high fat diet
G. Tallness
H. Oral contraceptive use, especially when young
I. Personal history of fibrocystic disease
J. Personal history of ovarian or endometrial cancer
K. Excessive alcohol consumption

Language can deceive. We have been led to believe that risk is the same as cause. Risk is not a cause of illness. Risk is a result of exposure to a hazard, as in the formula:

HAZARD + EXPOSURE = RISK

The highway is a risky place, and no one would believe that it is a safe place for children to play. We guard against risk of traffic injuries by keeping children (and adults) away from highways by erecting barriers, route planning, education, and laws. We still have the hazards of highway traffic, but have controlled and contained exposure, and thus limited risk.

Those with a sense of history will recall that fewer than 100 years ago diseases were spread from outhouses and sewage outfalls, and a major cause of illness came from contaminated water. Disease and death took its toll not only among the poor, but among the wealthy. It was to everyones' interest to bring the spread of infectious disease under control. This was accomplished by widespread *public* health programs. Public funds and public action were dedicated to control, disinfect, and clean sources of infection and to provide a clean supply of water. Thus public funds and public action secured benefit for the common good.

While we have largely eliminated the scourge of waterborne typhoid, we now have the epidemic of cancer that reaches into every neighborhood, every age group, and every segment of society. Massive public health efforts are again needed to stop this epidemic and prevent illness in others.

Without noticing, the public and indeed some scientists have been lulled into thinking that risk is the same as outcome. This message has come as well from some in the cancer establishment. Clearly, if either hazard or exposure is missing from the equation, there is no risk. What indeed are the risks for breast cancer and what are the implications? Taken one at time, they are discussed below.

Family History

The most often expressed "risk" is that of breast cancer in a "first-degree relative," that is a mother or sister. The occurrence of breast cancer within a family may indicate a genetic connection, but this is a factor in but 5 and no more than 10% of cases. A family history of breast cancer is one of the major criteria for inclusion into the tamoxifen experiment, the issues of which are discussed in Chapter 9. If one considers a genetic link only, one misses the other 90 to 95% of causes. These more critical factors include exposures common among family members who together may live near a contaminated source: downwind of an incinerator or nuclear power plant; a toxic dump site; a former military nuclear base; a plant discharging pollution into the air and water; an agricultural area. Nor is an inherited factor a major issue when generations eat food from the same contaminated source. Many family members have food consumption patterns in common, and may share work and exposure patterns.

Early Menarche

Since the turn of the century, menarche, the start of a girl's menstrual cycle, has occurred at younger and younger ages, with girls in the "developed" countries experiencing earlier menarche than girls in less developed countries. Early menarche reflects estrogenic action, the stimulus originating from a girl's own ovaries, or from foreign chemicals carried in her food and from her general environment. The synthetic estrogen diethylstilbestrol, widely used in meat animals in the fifties and sixties, produced premature sexual development in a girl, only five years old, when applied to the skin.[2] Six decades ago, it was demonstrated that premature puberty could be induced in test animals with a benzanthracene, a polycyclic aromatic compound[3] commonly found in organic fuels, oils, coal, coke, soot, and peat. Recognition of the estrogenic action of peat extracts formed the basis for the development of the stilbene drugs, including diethylstilbestrol (DES).

Late Menopause

Menopause, the cessation of a womans' menses, is the natural response to decreasing levels of hormones produced in her ovaries, and generally occurs around the age of 50. Normal cessation of menses may be delayed in the individual woman by hormones administered purposefully or taken inadvertently in her diet. Nonsurgical cessation of menses before the age of 45, or surgical removal of a woman's ovaries before age 40, confers a decreased risk of breast cancer. If a woman undergoes a hysterectomy, without removal of her ovaries, there is no change in her cancer risk.[4]

Late Childbirth and Pregnancy in General

Pregnancy is both a major stress and a major hormonal event. Seldom thought of, pregnancy is also a detoxification route for the mother, whereby chemicals stored in the mother's body are transferred to the fetus. Pregnancy later in life, particularly if delayed by the use of birth control pills, allows a period of time for hormonally active chemicals to accumulate in a woman's body.

Lesbians have been identified as having a higher risk of breast cancer. It is unlikely that sexual orientation plays any role in breast cancer, but that lesbians as a rule elect not to have children, and therefore do not experience the chemical mobilization and excretion aspects of pregnancy. Others have suggested the reason for more breast cancer among lesbians is alcohol abuse and greater obesity, but no studies have actually addressed these factors.

Identification of 280,965 women who had undergone a cumulative total of 370,715 induced abortions demonstrated no increase for breast cancer among those having the procedure before seven weeks of gestation.[5] The overall risk for breast cancer decreases with the number of full-term pregnancies. This follows biological principles in that toxic chemicals stored in the mother's body are transferred to the fetus and to the nursing infant with each pregnancy.

Breast Feeding

Nursing an infant has been demonstrated to lower breast cancer risk for the mother. The mother's milk becomes a detoxification route for the mother, while unfortunately, contaminating her infant when her milk contains toxic chemicals. Fat-soluble, hormonal substances are easily passed to the infant in the lipid-rich mother's milk. Transferred as well within the calcium-rich milk are radioactive isotopes such as strontium.

Conversely, from the biological point of view, it is difficult to believe that breast feeding when a woman is in her twenties is protective against the toxic exposures she receives between those years and when she is her fifties and sixties. No specific test data on this issue are available as of this writing.

The changing pattern of breast cancer is causing us to ask why some women develop breast cancer at younger and younger ages? Were these young women nursed two to four decades ago by mothers whose milk contained DES, DDT, PCBs, PBBs, dioxins, and radioactive isotopes? We know for certain that these chemicals are passed from mother to infant.

In the early 1970s in Michigan, there occurred a massive public health problem when animal feed was contaminated with polybrominated biphenyls (PBBs). An additive for animal feed, "Nutrimaster," had been accidentally replaced by a similar-looking product, a fire-retardant for plastics labeled "Firemaster." The latter contained PBBs. The PBB-contaminated feed was distributed to farmers who unwittingly fed it to their livestock and poultry. Realization of the health risks from the PBB contamination required the slaughter of thousands of cattle and poultry whose carcasses were buried in landfills.

Monitoring throughout the area revealed the PBB contamination to be widespread. This led the Michigan Department of Public Health to test the breast milk of 26 Michigan women. Twenty-two had detectable levels of PBBs, and all 22 resided in the lower peninsula of Michigan.[6] No PBBs were detected in 10 women from other states. In August 1976, the Michigan Department of Public Health issued a press release discouraging the testing of breast milk, stating "laboratory tests on an individual woman will not provide information to help her reach a decision on whether or not to breast feed."[7] This patronizing statement is a prime example of judgment imposed unilaterally upon the individual by medical, political, and economic forces. Withholding information and decisions from the affected person that are rightfully hers and could be used to protect her child is not only a health hazard, but an abridgement of personal rights.

By 1976, it was known that PBBs, like their chemical cousins the PCBs, held risks for toxicity to the embryo and newborn—that each were stored in tissues and excreted in milk, and each caused life-threatening effects.[8] Fifteen months later, testing showed PBB levels averaging from non-detectable to 1.22 parts per million (ppm), with levels as high as 92.66 ppm in the breast milk of women who had lived on quarantined farms.[9]

It is now 20-plus years since the initial PBB contamination. What has been the effect on Michigan women who were breast fed in those years? How many young women with breast cancer were nursed? And for how long? How many were raised on PBB-contaminated food?

For all women diagnosed with breast cancer, not only in Michigan but else-where, the least that should be done is to obtain a fat biopsy and assay for toxic chemicals such as PBBs, the related polychlorinated biphenyls (PCBs), the pesticide DDT and its breakdown product DDE, chlordane/heptachlor-related pesticides, and dioxins. My urging women to have tissue or blood assayed for toxic chemicals has been criticized on the basis of not having a "control" group with whom to compare. Think about that. These chemicals are entirely man-made. They are not found anywhere naturally, but occur as a result of contamination. There should be *no* detectable levels of these chemicals in anyone's bodies. Being completely foreign they serve no useful purpose in the body. All levels reflect contamination during the person's life.

Does the potential for contamination mean that women should not nurse their infants? The nutritional, nonallergenic, immunologic, and psychological benefits of uncontaminated breast milk to the infant far surpass any dairy or synthetic formula. But that does not answer the question whether to breast feed or not, because most women are unaware if they have been exposed to toxic chemicals and don't know if their breast milk is contaminated or not. Women concerned about exposing their infants have two options to determine if they carry significant contaminants. A woman can have a small amount of her body fat tested for foreign chemicals prior to delivery, or she can have her breast milk tested for contaminants soon after the birth of her infant in order to make an informed decision whether to nurse her child.

The procedure to have body fat tested involves removal of the equivalent of a teaspoon of fat from beneath the abdominal skin, either through a small incision, or via a large-bore suction-type device. The fat is placed in a glass container, frozen, and sent to a laboratory experienced in such testing. Unfortunately, most insurance programs do not cover such testing, even though it may be preventive medicine at its earliest.

In the event that toxic chemicals are detected, the safer decision for the infant's sake may be not to breast feed. And that decision raises a whole new set of problems: the plasticizers in nonglass baby bottles, natural estrogens in soy-based formula, and possible contaminants in cow's milk. Only when mother's milk can be protected from contamination will the breast-fed infant be spared the risk of such contamination, a risk rarely documented or measured.

Obesity and/or High Fat Diet

It appears that obesity confers not only an increased risk for breast cancer, but an increased risk for heart disease, hypertension, and degenerative arthritis. Is the obesity link to breast cancer due to toxic chemicals in our diet or to having a bountiful layer of fat on ones' body? Forming a reservoir, obese people have a greater volume of adipose tissue in which to store toxic chemicals than do thin people, and fatty foods are efficient carriers of carcinogenic and hormonal substances.[10]

More basically, do the hormonal chemicals in our diets promote both breast cancer and obesity? After all, hormones are administered to meat animals to promote growth and weight gain. Why should humans expect to not respond similarly to such chemical stimuli? This question and other hormone issues are explored in Chapter 6 of this book.

In addition to purposely administered hormonal growth agents, meat and dairy products may contain whatever chemicals the animals ate, were injected with, were applied to their bodies, or were used in their barns. Fish and shellfish may contain whatever toxins are in the water in which they grow, whether in the wild or in fish pond culture. Vegetable oils absorb whatever pesticides were applied to the plant and soil. Additionally, plastic containers and cans lined with plastics can leach contaminants into the food stored therein. Dr. Ana Soto and her colleagues at Tufts University in Boston found that the plastic, p-nonyl-phenol, leaching from polystyrene plastic tubes was estrogenic.[11] Dr. Soto's group also found that the pesticides endosulfan, toxaphene, and dieldrin have estrogenic effects when tested on human cells in the laboratory.[12] Foods variously contaminated with pesticides, industrial chemicals, and hormonally active substances may be eaten by the unaware family who thus accumulate a burden of toxic chemicals.

Unfortunately, freshwater fish appear to be among the most heavily contaminated of foods. A letter to physicians from the Michigan Department of Health (MDH) reported that fish from the Great Lakes and from a number of Michigan rivers were contaminated with PCBs in excess of the then existing Food and Drug Administration guideline of 5 ppm. The MDH communique stated: "As a precaution people should limit the amount of fish from these waters to no more than one meal per week—approximately one-half pound per meal. Children should avoid eating fish from this section of the [Kalamazoo] river. In addition, women who expect to bear children and women who are pregnant or nursing an infant should avoid eating these fish."[13]

One would question the wisdom of eating any amount of a contaminated food, given the biological activity and prolonged fat-storage of such chemicals as PCBs. More than likely, gradual accumulation of "small" amounts of toxic chemicals will reach a critical mass of harm.

Looking for a population uncontaminated by PCBs, Canadian researchers sought out the Inuit village on Broughton Island, in the north Atlantic. Unexpectedly and to the researchers' concern, they found the people of the island had the highest PCB levels of any human population. Only those exposed in industrial accidents exceeded them. The PCB source was the traditional Inuit diet: seal, polar bear, narwhals, and caribou, contaminated as

PCBs moved up the food-web.[14] Becoming a part of the food chain, PCBs contaminated the breast milk of the Arctic mothers.[15] The ultimate effects upon this population and their children nursed by these mothers are unknown.

In an unintended experiment during World War II, some 3 million Danish citizens were under blockade, deprived of meat and forced to live largely on bran, potatoes, greens, milk, and some butter. The result was a decline in deaths in men aged 25 to 63.[16] I am indebted to professor Herman Adlercreutz from the University of Helsinki for this information and for his data showing protection against cancer by eating a predominantly vegetarian diet, high in whole grains, soy, seeds, and nuts.[17] Soy plants are high in lignin and isoflavonoid glycosides that are converted by intestinal bacteria to hormone-like compounds with weak estrogenic and antioxidant activity. Unlike man-made fat-soluble xenoestrogens, these natural plant estrogens are water-soluble and influence a number of the body's protective mechanisms, including inhibition of cell proliferation and unwanted blood vessel growth, called angiogenesis.[18] Inhibition of angiogenesis is critical in stopping the growth of cancers, as was demonstrated in laboratory tests. Dr. Adlercreutz and his associates indicate these foods are "strong candidates for a role as natural cancer protective compounds."[19]

Clearly, the question of obesity and breast cancer involves more than good health practices. It is about not just how much we eat, but our actual diet, its source, and the purity of our food, free from purposeful and unintended contamination.

Tallness

Tallness, greater than 68 inches, was associated with increased breast cancer, diagnosed in both young and older women.[20] A parallel issue of large size and obesity in humans is the use of hormonal agents to raise animals for meat. If the current animal drugs are transferred to the consumer in meat and dairy products, as was the growth-promoting chemical diethylstilbestrol (DES), then there is no reason why humans, exposed to the current anabolic drugs, will not grow taller and gain weight as do farm animals dosed with these drugs.

Since the ban on using DES for raising animals for food, there has been little information provided to the consumer about other steroid products administered to livestock. As of 1995, the Food and Drug Administration allows the use of implanted hormonal agents for raising beef cattle. These include the female hormones estradiol and progesterone; norgestomet, a synthetic progestin; the male hormone testosterone; and the synthetic anabolic steroids zeranol and trenbolone. Growth agents that do not have to be implanted include the progestin melengestrol that can be added to the animals' feed. None of the hormonal agents require a withdrawal period prior to slaughter. Indeed, the FDA does not require mandatory recording of medication or treatment of meat animals.[21]

In dairy cows and veal calves, no withdrawal period prior to marketing is required during the use of estradiol, progesterone, or the synthetics norgestomet and zeranol. Do these chemicals pass into the milk supply, and into our cheese and yogurt? Few data are available to the public. Moreover, correspondence with one supplier of vegetable oils indicates that no testing for leaching of plastic from containers into the oil products has been done.[22]

So again, what factors are involved in increased body size and weight? We must assume from the evidence that nutrition and hormones play a role in growth and obesity for humans as well as for farm animals, and may be factors contributing to the development of breast cancer.

Ovarian or Endometrial Cancer

There is evidence that women and their close relatives who develop ovarian and endometrial cancer are at increased risk for breast cancer. All these malignancies are under hormonal influence, and the links are confirmed in studies linked to DES, tamoxifen, and post-menopausal hormones. The scientific ramifications of these chemicals are discussed in detail in Chapters 6, 7, 8, and 9 of this volume.

Fibrocystic Breast Disease

At this time, it is unknown if women with benign fibrocystic changes in their breasts are at increased risk for breast cancer. A lump, felt by a woman and biopsied to rule out cancer, often is found to have fibrocystic changes. These women may become more aware of breast changes and have more mammographic studies, increasing their exposure to radiation. Whether the prime factor is the fibrocystic change or increased numbers of mammograms, the final outcome is still unknown, but bears careful scrutiny.

Oral Contraceptive Use

Oral contraceptive use, especially in young women, has been reported to increase the incidence of breast cancer,[23] especially after prolonged use of the products.[24] Oral contraceptive products, developed earlier in the 1960s and 1970s, contained higher levels of both estrogen and progesterone components than the current products. The ultimate findings of incidence and distribution of breast cancer, connected to these products, will not be revealed until women who used them pass menopause. Giving little comfort is adenocarcinoma of the cervix, greatest after 12 years of hormonal contraceptive use, confirming further the effects of hormonal agents upon the female organs of reproduction.

Excessive Alcohol Consumption

It has been proposed that alcohol consumption raises estrogen concentration, but studies are preliminary and more research is needed. Rather than a direct carcinogenic effect, ethanol exerts its action by interfering with the liver's metabolism of foreign chemicals, including estrogens. Given the number and amounts of pesticides used on grapes and grain, the building blocks of wine and liquor, perhaps the culprit may not prove to be alcohol, but contaminants therein. Another facet ripe for study.

THESE RISKS IN PERSPECTIVE

What is the message running through all of these "risks"? Hormones, hormones, and hormones. Hormones of the wrong kind, hormones too soon in a girl's life, hormones for too many years in a woman's life, too many chemicals with hormonal action, and too great a total hormonal load. Another key is the *kind* of hormones, the foreign chemicals.

Conflicting with the finding of decreased breast cancer risk after the ovaries are removed is the finding that the natural hormones produced by a woman do not result in a breast cancer increase.[26] Should we then consider that the increasing incidence of breast cancer is linked to the overload of foreign hormonal agents?

Another aspect that gives lie to the genetic "risk" issue is an increase in breast cancer when women migrate from a low-incidence area to one of a high incidence. Asian migrants who have lived a decade or more in the West have an

80% increased risk of developing breast cancer compared to more recent arrivals.[27] This shift gives credence to findings that environmental factors are the major culprits. Change of residence often carries a marked change in lifestyle, major components of which are diet and environment.

OTHER RISK FACTORS— AVOIDABLE IF KNOWN

Collectively, some risk factors are very troubling, not only in the United States, but worldwide. A number of these factors have been identified. The questions are: Do we have the will and the ability to change both our individual and institutional prejudices and practices? Can we interrupt the political and economic forces that have the environment and human health firmly in its grip?

Earlier in our history we achieved control of hazardous, unproven, untested, and dangerous drugs, such as arsenic-containing "tonics" and other nostrums. Regulations under the Food and Drug Act stopped the use of birth-defect-producing thalidomide; curtailed the unwarranted use of the antibiotic Chloromycetin (chloramphenicol) linked to the fatal blood condition aplastic anemia; withdrew approval of the anti-diabetes drug, DBI (phenformin);[28] removed the anti-inflammatory drug, Zomax (zomepirac); and curtailed the use of silicone breast implants, and other hazardous products.

Other hazards, not definitively proved, but implicated in cancer growth, have maintained acceptance in the marketplace. Canadian researchers demonstrated enhanced cancer growth in mice given daily *human-equivalent* doses of three commonly used antihistamines.[29] These are loratidine, astemizole, and hydroxyzine, sold as Schering Corporation's Claritin; Histamil from Janssen Pharmaceutica; and Atarax from the Roerig division of Pfizer Corporation. Claritin and Histamil are advertised directly to the public in newspaper supplements and on television, the former offering a five dollar rebate coupon to the *customer*.

Two years previously, the same Canadian researchers described promotion of malignant growth in rodents with antidepressant drugs, at *clinically relevant doses*.[30] These drugs included amitriptyline, marketed as Elavil, and sold by Stuart Pharmaceuticals, "A Business unit of ICI," and fluoxetine, better recognized as Prozac, marketed by Dista Products Company, a division of Eli Lilly.[31]

These drugs bind to growth-regulating receptors inside of cells associated with antiestrogen binding sites. When given to rats primed with a known carcinogen, the animals developed breast tumors in a shortened period of time. Compared to controls, the tumor frequency was increased greater than two-fold in the antidepressant-treated rats.[32] A report from University of Maryland's Department of Epidemiology and Preventive Medicine shows tumor promotion with amitriptyline and fluoxetine (Prozac).[33] As of the publishing date of this book, it is unknown what course, if any, the FDA is taking on these issues.

Ordinarily, in humans and animals alike, breast milk is formed only after a female has given birth to an offspring. Certain chemicals, however, are able to promote breast development and milk release even in virgin animals. In the late 1950s, I worked in the laboratory of Dr. Joseph Meites at Michigan State University, where lactation was produced in virgin animals with the drug chlorpromazine. This drug is prescribed for a number of psychiatric conditions and marketed worldwide under many different trade names. It is sold in the United States as Thorazine. Physiologically, any stimulus to the release of prolactin, be it cessation of pregnancy or chemically initiated, has the potential to cause growth oo breast cells. That cellular growth is normal as occurs after the birth of a child. In the absence of pregnancy and breast feeding, those stimulated cells may be transformed into cancer.

According to the current manufacturer, SmithKline Beecham, indications for use of Thorazine include psychosis, nausea, and vomiting, "relief of restlessness and apprehension before surgery," and "severe behavioral problems in children." After stating "tissue culture experiments indicate that approximately one-third of human breast cancers are prolactin-dependent in vitro, a fact of potential importance if the prescribing of these drugs is contemplated in a patient with a previously detected breast cancer," and continuing, "an increase in mammary neoplasms has been found in rodents after chronic administration of neuroleptic drugs," it concludes "neither clinical nor epidemiological studies conducted to date, however, have shown an association between chronic administration of these drugs and mammary tumorigenesis; the available evidence is considered too limited to be conclusive at this time."[34]

How many women are questioned about use of such drugs? Are their physicians even aware that there may be a connection? Is this why the available evidence is "considered too limited to be conclusive at this time," because no one thought about it?

Review of the chemical structure of chlorpromazine shows a remarkable similarity to the structure of dioxins (Figure 3.1), where nitrogen and sulfur molecules are substituted for oxygen molecules in the central ring, leading one to question if there is a similar mechanism in action. . . . I could find no definitive answer.

Considering that chlorpromazine has been available since the patent was issued to Rhone Poulenc in 1952, one has to question why patients receiving this drug have not been followed with diligence; why there has been no FDA alert; why no registry has been established; and why available evidence is so limited. Countless patients have been given this drug. What has been their fate? Men patients treated with Thorazine complained when they developed unwanted breast growth. Are they among the men now developing breast cancer?

We do not know if any of these psychoactive drugs, given to women, depressed about learning they have breast cancer, have accelerated tumor growth. In general, women develop depression more often than men, and are frequently treated with antidepression drugs. What role, if any, these antidepression and antihistamine drugs play in accelerating breast cancer is unknown. Prozac and Elavil are related in action, blocking chemical messengers released from mast cells, and binding to special liver cells, called P450 enzyme receptors.[35]

Two sales representatives from Eli Lilly, the manufacturer of Prozac, distributed promotional materials at a "National Depression Awareness Day" program at a Bethesda, Maryland, high school.[36] There is something at odds

Figure 3.1
Chlorpromazine and mono-chloro-dioxin

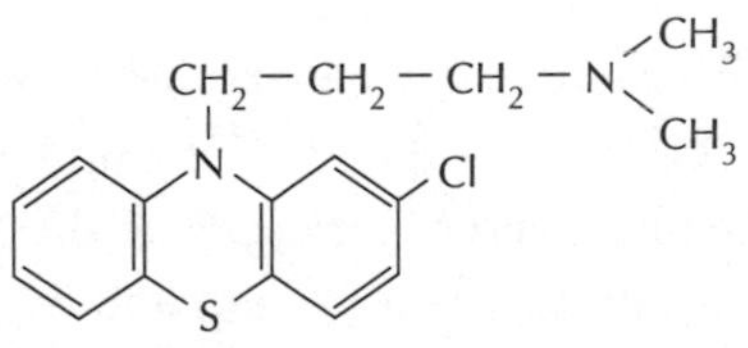

CHLORPROMAZINE

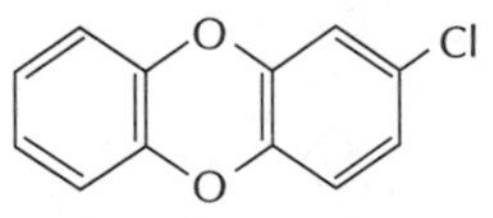

MONO-CHLORO-DIOXIN

in this message to our youth. Does Nancy Reagan's slogan "Say no to drugs" apply only to street drugs? Mood swings among teens are not a recent phenomenon. They are part of reaching maturity and learning to cope with stresses and emotions without resorting to drugs—be they street drugs or prescription drugs.

Inquiring into *past* medication use is not a common medical practice. Such information-gathering should become routine for all physicians treating cancer patients. Given that drug-free, alternative therapies are available for many conditions, one should argue for caution, or at least patient warning, before prescribing drugs with significant biological effects.

Education is at the heart of every prevention program. Every woman receiving a prescription for any of these products should be informed in writing of side effects and adverse findings. It is hoped that the breast cancer activist organizations will support not only this effort, but promote questionnaires concerning past medication use for every oncology treatment facility. The number of women with breast cancer who were prescribed any of these drugs, and what their effects were, is simply unknown.

Change in practice is extremely difficult if hazards carry liability for harm, bear costs for cleanup, or result in loss of profit by eliminating a product or process. It is only through knowledge that "risk" can be separated from hazard and exposure, and pressure can be brought to change our practices. For without change in business as usual, we can expect the breast cancer epidemic to continue to escalate.

REDUCING RISK BY REDUCING ABSORBED CHEMICAL LOAD

A treatment regimen proposed for patients with high levels of fat-soluble toxins in their bodies has been developed. First and foremost is to eliminate the intake of toxic chemicals and pesticides from the diet and water. Ridding the body of these toxins utilizes heat (sauna) and exercise to increase mobilization of chemicals from fat stores, and once mobilized, to speed excretion in the urine and feces. Some programs have demonstrated a lessening of the chemical burden in a number of patients.

Two notable programs are those administered by Dr. William Rea and his colleagues in Dallas, Texas, and Dr. Fox and associates in Fall River, Nova Scotia, Canada. Some aspects of detoxification programs have been under attack from various quarters, notably attorneys defending toxic chemical cases, the insurance industry, and some physicians. While cost of such residence programs are a problem, it must be argued that encouragement and support should be given to programs that lessen the chemical load borne by seriously ill patients. Training in methods of detoxification should be developed at local centers and made available for low cost for those who need the treatment.

Most institutional environmental detoxification programs are neither simple nor inexpensive. But until it is accepted public policy to prevent contamination, prevent illness, and provide remediation, there will remain a need for detoxification mechanisms for people already contaminated.

For those who do not know their toxic chemical load, but want to minimize any effect and promote prevention, we know that exercise and heat increase mobilization of fat-soluble toxins. Therefore one does not require a formal program to understand the need for vigorous exercise; the benefits of a high-fiber diet to enhance bowel function; and the prudence of eating a toxin-free diet and drinking uncontaminated water.

In our convoluted world, it is acceptable to perform on patients experimental surgical, drug, and medical procedures that are painful, costly, and of dubious value, while attacking some programs designed to ameliorating the chemical burden. If prevention of contamination were first in consideration, we would not need remedial decontamination of ourselves and of our environment.

RISKS, BENEFITS, COSTS, AND ASSESSMENTS

This author was a member an advisory committee for the EPA's Toxic Substances Control Act and served on a Risk-Benefit subcommittee. It became apparent that risks and benefits do not accrue to the same entity. Typically, producers of products benefited enormously from sales, while those purchasing and using the products bore whatever the risks.

In the early 1980s the risk-benefit language changed, and benefit became cost, and Risk-Cost analysis became popular. Technocrats then argued that costs of cleanup, costs for change in technology, and costs of prevention exceeded risks. Therefore risks then became "acceptable." More recently the pendulum has not swung, but stuck in place: industry and government bureaucrats perform "Risk Analysis" obscuring any mention of who benefits and who is at risk. Risk analysis aims to minimize problems by presenting risks as so many sick or dead spread over a million of the population.

Because most of us have difficulty with the concept of a million of anything, the asserted risk numbers become unreal. This twist of logic aims to spread the idea of risk over the entire population. In reality, only those exposed to a hazard are at risk, be the risk chemicals, nuclear radiation, drugs, traffic, or any other entity. The next step in bureaucratese has been to institutionalize the idea of "acceptable risk." Acceptable to whom?

Simply put, hazards are everywhere. But that is not a reason for despair. Hazards linked to breast cancer have not existed in such numbers and amounts until recent times, essentially the past 40 to 50 years. That means that risk is not inevitable: with knowledge and effort, pressure can and must be brought to eliminate and control these hazards and reduce our risks. Until that is done, *we all are at risk, every woman, indeed everyone.* Learning the true nature of risk has been obscured. We have not come to terms with the factors that comprise risk. In the face of being redundant,

$$RISK = HAZARD + EXPOSURE$$

HISTORY REPEATS ITSELF

> It is a well established fact, that diseases are not confined to the localities where they originate, but widely diffuse their poisonous miasma. Hence, though the poor may fall in greater numbers because of their nearer proximity to the causes of disease, yet the rich who inhabit the splendid squares and spacious streets . . . often become the victims of the same disorders which afflict their poorer brethren.[37]

The above was written in regard to the wretched sanitary conditions existing in New York City in the 1800s. It is apparent that preserving public health and promoting the common good benefits all of society. This concept is applicable to every known and proposed risk for breast cancer. If we are to prevent cancer and promote human health we must protect our common environment.

In the final analysis, if we consider that the "traditional" risk factors account for perhaps 30% of breast cancers, we are left with the fact that **more than 70%** of women who develop breast cancer have **none** of the "traditional" factors linked to breast cancer "risk." When we understand this, we can stop blaming women for being tall or overweight, and stop laying blame on our inheritance.

REFERENCES

1. Fulghum, R. All I Really Need to Know I Learned in Kindergarten. Villard Books, Random House, New York. 1986.
2. Whittle, C., Lyell, A. Precocity in a girl aged 5: due to stilbestrol inunction. Proc. Royal Soc. Med. 41(11): 36, 1948.
3. Cook, J. W., Dodds, E. C., Hewett, C. L., Lawson, W. The oestrogenic activity of some condensed-ring compounds in relation to their other biological activates. Proc. Royal Soc. 104: 272–286, 1033/34.
4. Crosby, W. H., What are my chances of getting breast cancer? J. Amer. Med. Assoc. 238(4): 345–346, 1977.
5. Melbye, M., Wohlfahrt, J., Olsen, J. H., Frisck, M., Westergaard, T., Helwig-Larsen, K., Andersen, P. K. Induced abortion and the risk of breast cancer. New Engl. J. Med. 336(2): 81–85, 1997.
6. Feinberg, L., Miller, R. W. Pollutants in breast milk, PBBs: The ladies' milk is not for burning. J. Pediatr. 90(3): 510–512, 1977.
7. Reizen, M. S., Director, Michigan Department of Health. Letter to Michigan Physicians. 2 pages. August 26, 1976.
8. Sherman, J. D. Polybrominated biphenyl exposure and human cancer: report of a case and public health implications. Toxicol. Indust. Health 7(3): 197–205, 1991. In this paper, I report virtually unchanging fat levels of PBBs over an 11-year period, in a person dying of cancer.
9. Reizen, M. S., Director Michigan Department of Public Health. Dear Doctor letter. 2 pages. November 29, 1977.
10. Beer, A. E., Billingham, R. E. Adipose tissue, a neglected factor in aetiology of breast cancer? Lancet. p. 296. August 5, 1978.
11. Soto, A. M., Justicia, H., Wray, J. W., Sonnenschein, C. p-nonyl-phenol: An estrogenic xenobiotic released from "modified" polystyrene. Environ. Health Perspect. 92: 167–173, 1991.
12. Soto, A. M., Chung, K. L., Sonnenschein, C. The pesticides endosulfan, toxaphene and dieldrin have estrogenic effects on human estrogen-sensitive cells. Environ. Health Perspect. 102(4): 380–383, 1994.
13. Reizen, M. S., Director Michigan Department of Health. Dear Doctor letter. 2 pages November 29, 1977.
14. Colborn, T., Dumanoski, D., Myers, J. P. Our Stolen Future. Dutton. New York. pp. 106–107, 1996.
15. Dewailly, E., Nantel, A., Weber, J. Meyer, F. High levels of PCBs in breast milk of Inuit women from the Arctic Quebec. Bull. Environ. Contam. Toxicol. 43: 641–646, 1989.
16. Hindhede, M. The effect of food restriction during war on mortality in Copenhagen. J. Amer. Med. Assoc. 74(6): 381–382, 1920.
17. Adlercreutz, H. Western diet and Western diseases: some hormonal and biochemical mechanisms and associations. Scand. J. Clin. Lab. Invest. 50 Suppl. 201: 3–23, 1990.

18. Fotsis, T., Pepper, M., Adlercreutz, H., Hase, T., Montesano, R., Schweigerer, L. Genistein, a dietary ingested isoflavonoid, inhibits cell proliferation and in vitro angiogenesis. J. Nutrit. 125: 790S–797S, 1995.

19. Adlercreutz, C. H. T., Goldin, B. R., Gorbach, S. L., Hockerstedt, K. A. V., Watanabe, S., Hamalainen, E. K., Markkanen, M. H., Makela, T. U., Wahala, K. T., Hase, T. A., Fotsis, T. Soybean phytoestrogen intake and cancer risk. J. Nutrit. 125: 757S–770S, 1995.

20. Brinton, L. A., Swanson, C. A. Height and weight at various ages and risk of breast cancer. Ann. Epidemiol. 2: 597–609, 1992.

21. U.S. FDA. Center for Veterinary Medicine. CVM Memo. Drug Use Guide: Beef Cattle. 12 pp., June 1995.

22. Pet Foods, Inc., 1-page letter dated April 8, 1994.

23. Pike, M. C., Henderson, B. E., Krailo, M. D., Duke, A., Roy, S. Breast cancer in young women and use of oral contraceptives: possible modifying effect of formulation and age at use. Lancet. ii: 926–930, 1983.

24. Chilvers, C. Oral contraceptives and Cancer. Lancet. 344: 1378–1379, 1994.

25. Ursin, G., Peters, R. K., Henderson, B. E., d'Ablaing III, G., Monroe, K. R., Pike, M. C. Oral contraceptive use and adenocarcinoma of cervix, Lancet. 344: 1390–1394, 1994.

26. Helzlsouer, K. J., Alberg, A. J., Bush, T. L., Longcope, C. A prospective study of endogenous hormones and breast cancer. Cancer Detect. Prev. 18(2): 79–85, 1994.

27. Ziegler, R. G., Hoover, R. N., Pike, M. C., Hildesheim, A., Nomura, A. M. Y., West, D. W., Wu-Williams, A. H., Kolonel, L. N., Horn-Ross, P. L., Rosenthal, J. F., Hyer, M. B. Migration patterns and breast cancer risk in Asian-American women. J. Nat. Cancer Inst. 85(22): 1819–1827, 1993.

28. Bigelow-Sherman, J. D., Foa, P. P. Lactic acidosis, diabetes mellitus and the biguanide compounds. Acta Diabetologica Latina. 6:50–522, 1969.

29. Brandes, L. J., Warrington, R. C., Arron, R. J., Bogdanovic, R. P., Fang, W., Queen, G. M., Stein, D. A., Tong, J., Zaborniak, C. L. F., LaBelle, F. S. Enhanced cancer growth in mice administered daily human-equivalent doses of some H1-antihistamines: Predictive in vitro correlates. J. Nat. Cancer Inst. 86(10): 770–775, 1994.

30. Brandes, L. J., Lorne, J., Arron, R., Bogdanovic, P., Tong, J., Zaborniak, C., Hogg, G. Wassington, R., Fang, W., LaBelle, F. Stimulation of malignant growth in rodents by antidepressant drugs at clinically relevant doses. Cancer Res. 52(13): 3796–3800, 1992.

31. As of November 1993, it was estimated that there were 10 million users of Prozac or similar products. Four years after Prozac was marketed, it brought over $1 billion in sales to the manufacturer, Eli Lilly. Thompson, T. The wizard of Prozac. Washington Post. pp. F-1,5. November 11, 1993.

32. Brandes et al. Op.

33. Stolley, P. D., Zahm, S. H. Nonhormonal drugs and cancer. Environ. Health Perspect. 103(8): 191–196, 1995.

34. Physician's Desk Reference. Medical Economics Data Production Co., Montvale, N.J., 49th edition, pp. 2408–2410, 1995.

35. Nemecek, S. Backfire—Could Prozac and Elavil promote tumor growth? Sci. Amer. 22–23, September 1994.

36. Day., K. Depression awareness—or a Prozac pitch? Washington Post. pp. F-1,2. January 18, 1995.

37. New York Public Library. The History and Politics of Trash in New York City from 1840–1920. Exhibition, November 12, 1994 through February 25, 1995.

4

BREAST CANCER DIAGNOSIS
MAMMOGRAPHIC AND OTHER METHODS

Breast cancer is all too common, and there are few reliable methods for detecting the disease in its early stage. Experience shows that most cancers are found by the woman herself. Feeling a mass or having a mammogram are the currently recommended methods. Either way, the abnormality has to be large enough to be felt or seen. Another method of screening is available, and that is thermography, a heat-sensing technique, but it is not well-developed in the United States, nor widely available.

To date, in contrast to the specific blood test for prostate cancer (PSA or prostate specific antigen), there are no reliable blood or urine tests reflecting a change in the body's physiology that would signal a developing breast malignancy. Hence, regular self-examination still remains the major screening tool. Women still having their menses experience an increased fullness in their breasts prior to menstruation, so the best time to examine ones' breasts is at the end of ones' menstrual period. These examinations should be done regularly, every month. For women past menopause, it helps to mark the calendar to set a regular time for beast self-examination. It is important for every woman to become familiar with the topography of her own breasts, and to be able to detect any change in the texture of her breast tissue. Examination should include not only breast tissue, but ones' axillae (armpits) as well. For some women, the first sign of a breast lesion is an enlarged lymph node in the axilla.

A yearly thorough breast examination by a physician or nurse practitioner trained in the technique of breast examination is very important. Breast and gynecological examinations should be done yearly. The latter should include a Pap* smear and pelvic examination. These two procedures are able to detect two major causes of sickness and death in women. It is reassuring to know that most insurance programs now cover the cost of mammographic and Pap tests, although this was not always so, and obviously counter to the precept of preventive medicine.

Dr. Rosalie Bertell is a Catholic Nun with the International Institute of Concern for Public Health in Toronto. She is a brilliant gray-haired woman and a world expert in the hazards of ionizing radiation. Dr. Bertell maintains that nurses trained in breast examinations, and who do this exclusively, are as good as radiographic mammography for picking up small tumors. An additional advantage of the nurses is that they can teach women how to do self-examination between professional examinations.

In order to improve the quality of care for women, the state of California provides a state-mandated publication called Breast Cancer Treatment Booklet in both English and Spanish. State law requires that physicians give this booklet to all patients before they perform a biopsy or treatment for breast disease, and to note receipt of the booklet in the patient's chart. Additionally, the California Department of Health Services has a continuing education curriculum to improve early detection of breast cancer. This guide is available as Clinical Breast Examination: Proficiency and Risk Management.[1]

Mammography, a radiological procedure, is a matter of concern, not the least of which is that it is not a preventive measure, but one of detection. Mammography involves exposure to x-irradiation, an established factor in cancer causation. Standard mammography, the current practice to "prevent" breast cancer, has become in reality, a program of early diagnosis, aiming for early treatment. The press touts mammographic screening to prevent breast cancer. In reality, screening has no effect upon prevention. Actual prevention means eliminating factors that cause cancer in the first place.

Mammography employs an x-ray image of each breast, allowing a physician to look for calcification, vascular abnormalities, masses, and other anatomic findings. Special equipment is now available whereby each breast is x-rayed after being compressed top-to-bottom, and then laterally. As the mammographic technique has improved, and as facilities upgrade their

*Named after Dr. George Papanicolaou, the developer of the cytological procedure to detect abnormal cells in a smear of uterine and cervical secretions.

equipment, the doses of radiation delivered to a woman have decreased. But this has not been always so, and so radiation doses have varied over time and from facility to facility.

Dr. John Gofman, physician and doctor of nuclear and physical medicine, notes that mammography involves not only financial expense, but more importantly, exposure to potentially harmful radiation. Between a rock and a hard place, as we might say. In his book, *X-rays: Health Effects of Common Exams,*[2] Dr. Gofman explains a method to calculate the radiation dosage from mammography, with the dose dependent upon the kind of mammographic equipment used and thickness of a woman's breasts. "The risks apply to women with breast of average size: 6 cm thick (approximately 2 3/8 inches) under compression."[3] The current type of examination employs a film-screen mode using a molybdenum target x-ray tube. Now obsolete in the United States was a technique that used a xeroradiography tungsten target x-ray tube. While the xerox method appeared to provide better definition, it delivered a higher dose of radiation. Mammography, by either method, indeed by any method that employs x-irradiation, increases the risk of breast cancer, increasing with each cumulative dose.

Dr. John Gofman provided Table 4.1, adapted from his book, *Preventing Breast Cancer.*[4] He emphasized the following basics:

- Examination done at an accredited mammography facility.
- Mean glandular x-ray dose per view = 0.1 rad (0.1 centiGray, cGy).
- There are two views of each breast per examination.
- Combined mean glandular dose to each breast = 0.2 rad (0.2 cGy).
- Unrepaired damage to genes from x-rays accumulates.

Therefore the risk from multiple mammograms is the sum of the risk from each individual exam.

Dr. Gofman explained that the typical exam supposedly gives a total dose of 0.2 rad, but that regulations permit a mean glandular dose three times higher (up to 0.6 rad total dose per exam); therefore every risk estimate could be three times higher. Mammograms that turn out to be "false positive" often result in additional x-ray procedures and risk. Some women will be at lower risk per exam, and others at higher risk. There is presently no way to identify which women are most vulnerable to x-ray-induced cancer. In all the examples above, an individual's chance of never getting mammogram-induced cancer far exceeds the risk of getting mammogram-induced cancer. Still, low risk is not "imaginary" or "hypothetical."

Table 4.1
Mammography: An Individual's Estimated Risk that the Examination Itself Will Cause Radiation-Induced Cancer

Age at Exam	Risk of Mammogram-Induced Breast Cancer
Any age in 30–34 range	1 exam: 1 chance in about 1100 5 exams: 5 chances/1100, or 1 chance/220
Age at exam 35–49 range	1 exam: 1 chance in about 1900 10 exams: 10 chances/1900, or 1 chance/190
Age at exam 50–64 range	1 exam: 1 chance in about 2000 15 exams: 15 chances/2000, or 1 chance in 133

These risks refer to incidence: mortality is approximately four times lower. Dr. Gofman said he has no data on exposure beyond age 64 at this time.

Should a woman not have mammograms? That is a difficult question to answer. Dr. Rosalie Bertell cautions against the use of mammographic screening programs, maintaining that more cancers are caused by radiating population groups. She cites a study of 50,000 Canadian women: Of those between the ages of 40 and 49 who had mammograms, 44 developed breast cancer; of those who did not have mammograms, 29 developed the disease. While the study needs additional analysis, Dr. Bertell maintains that "no level of mammography exposure can be presumed safe, particularly for females under 55 years of age."[5] The problem of a false positive can lead to additional x-ray exposure for confirmation of the original findings, as well as unnecessary surgery. Dr. Bertell urges, however, if a woman feels a mass in her breast, should she have a mammogram or elect to have a biopsy without delay.

When we go for a mammogram, it is important to be informed and to ask questions of the physician, the technician, and of the facility to determine that one is getting the most accurate of diagnostic procedures with the least amount of radiation exposure. If our questions are not answered satisfactorily, or not answered at all, we must be persistent, and if necessary, get information from State or Provincial Regulatory agencies. Most states require inspection, calibration, and certification of x-ray facilities. It is not only in the United States, but in Canada as well, where radiation dosages have been demonstrated to vary by several orders of magnitude.[6]

Dr. Edward Webster, radiation physicist from the Massachusetts General Hospital, commented: "When a woman arrives at a doctor's office for a mammogram, she has no way of knowing whether she is getting three hundred or three thousand millirads"[7] [of radiation].

Until October 1994, there was still no standard for mammography certification. Passage by Congress of the Mammography Quality Standards Act
(MQSA) mandates the FDA to set standards of compliance for facilities
covering:

- Quality assurance and control
- Radiological equipment
- Personnel qualifications of technicians who perform mammographies;
  physicians who interpret films; and physicists who monitor equipment
- Record keeping and report transmission[8]

The simple measure of informing a woman of her mammogram results,
in writing, is now part of the new guidelines.[9] This was not the previous
practice. As of 1996, more than one-third of mammographic facilities
seeking accreditation had failed on the first attempt.[10] It is hoped that these
guidelines may eliminate some concerns, and with care, may eliminate
some serious hazards. By utilization of modern techniques, mammographic
radiation exposure has been decreased by 10-fold over the past 25 years.

Early enthusiasm for mammography was spurred on by the American
Cancer Society, in conjunction with the National Cancer Institute, which in
the early 1970s established a program of free mammograms at 27 centers. By
1976, John C. Bailar III, then editor of the NCI Journal, wrote: "The possible
benefits of mammography have received more emphasis in the clinical literature than have its defects," adding "mammography may eventually cause
more deaths from breast cancer than it prevents."[11] Then came studies
showing little improvement in survival for women younger than age of 50
diagnosed with breast cancer. Twenty-two years later, Dr. Bailar, who had left
the NCI in frustration, found that the age-adjusted death rate for cancer was
6.0% higher in 1994 than it was in 1970. He wrote: "The war against cancer is
far from over. . . . The most promising approach in the control of cancer is a
national commitment to prevention, with a concomitant rebalancing of the
focus and funding of research."[12]

Despite the increasing cancer rate, in 1987 the ACS reversed its earlier
recommendation against mammography for women younger than 50, and
urged a "baseline" mammogram at age 35, followed by mammograms every
other year until age 40 to 50 and every year after that. By 1994, both the
National Cancer Institute and the American College of Physicians
recommended beginning mammograms at age 50 and every two years after
that. Still, physicians and medical providers (read insurance companies) have

differed over the need and optimum schedule for mammographic examination.

While mammography can show a tumor up to two years before it can be palpated, and detect 85 to 90% of tumors in women older than 50, it still fails to find between 10 and 15% of breast tumors.[13] That was the word in 1994. By 1998, a team of five women and one man from the University of Washington in Seattle and Harvard surveyed 2400 women who had mammograms over a 10-year period. They found that one-third had falsely abnormal mammograms. These women then required an additional evaluation—ultrasound, biopsy, and/or additional mammogram.[14] Thus, we find, even in major medical centers, that the prime method advocated to detect breast cancer is far from acceptable. Moreover, in women younger than 50, the chance of missing a malignant lesion is much higher.

If survival is determined by diagnosing and treating breast cancers when they are small, have not spread, and with no lymph node involvement, isn't the message a mixed one? Some studies show poorer survival of women diagnosed with breast cancer at younger ages. This may not simply be failure of mammography, but more aggressive tumors, or estrogen-dependent tumors, in keeping with the active hormonal state of younger women.

Then, too, economics may have influenced NCI's recommendations. It appears there may be two tiers of care: "the top tier driven by the advice of doctor to patient, the bottom tier driven by cost-conscious national policy." One senior Clinton administration official was quoted as saying, disapprovingly, "that the cost of providing every American woman in her 40s with a mammogram would run at least $2 billion a year."[15]

Various other procedures are being developed, including nuclear magnetic resonance, doppler ultrasound, echography, and thermography, but each has limitations. Considering the carcinogenic risks from radioactive isotope releases into the environment and the cumulative risk from mammographic radiation exposures, an alternative diagnostic procedure is needed. One of the most promising is thermography, a technique whereby infrared sensitive detectors are used to measure heat emitted through the skin and then to observe differences in temperature distribution in each of a woman's breasts.

Thermography has found wide use in the field of rheumatic and occlusive vascular diseases, measuring increased heat in inflamed joints, or decreased heat, as a result of decreased blood flow in limbs with occluded arteries. The technique has not been as successful in the field of mammography for a number of reasons. Some of the reasons are technical, some economic, and some political. Among technical reasons are the same as requirements for radiographic mammography: standardization of procedures, quality assurance, training, and a factor unique to thermography, definition of a "normal" breast.

Most pre-menopausal women are aware of breast changes coincident with changes with their menstrual cycle. These changes result in differences in thermographic readings. A positive thermographic diagnosis is based upon a difference in temperature between the two breasts. These differences reflect blood flow, inflammation, metabolism, and biological rhythms. Compared to traditional x-ray mammography that depicts anatomic structure, thermography measures functional status, that is, the actual physiological processes going on in the breast at the time of the thermographic examination.

A new safe screening procedure utilizes a temperature-sensitive soft pad that fits over the entire breast. The woman waits for 15 minutes, then removes the pad, which displays the pattern of temperature. If an area is significantly hotter, a more traditional mammography can be done for additional diagnosis.

Combining these two techniques, radiographic and thermographic, raises the rate of detection above that offered by either technique alone.[16] Significantly, women with a positive breast thermogram and a negative radiological mammogram had an 11% higher probability of developing cancer within the following 5 years than those with a negative heat study.[17,18] Abnormal thermograms were associated with tumors displaying a greater proportion of cells showing a proliferating DNA (biologically active) phase.[19] The findings may reflect faster growing tumors, with poorer prognosis, as associated with increased mitotic index and a positive thermogram.[20] Logically then, it appears that thermography may prove life-saving for women by its ability to detect fast-growing, aggressive tumors.

As with many techniques and products, thermology had its beginnings in military applications. When such engineering applications lost defense markets, the developers looked for new applications, and cancer detection seemed a natural development. Unfortunately, early thermology lacked both specificity (that is, failure to find a cancer or high false-negative rate) and sensitivity (the ability to detect small, early changes) as offered by radiological mammography. Both sensitivity and specificity approached that of physical examination and traditional mammography[21] in the hands of some investigators, but this was not universally so.

Twenty year ago, the Joint Working Group from the National Cancer Institute and the American Cancer Society concluded that "thermography does not appear to be suitable as a substitute for mammography for routine screening" and recommend discontinuation as a routine procedure, while it stressed "high priority be given to [such] studies." It noted that "thermography has no radiation risk and is less costly than mammography, and continued developmental work on this procedure, as well as other techniques suitable for screening, is needed."[22] But effort and money did not follow the NCI/ACS words.

Initially, thermology came under the umbrella of radiologists, specialists in structure not accustomed to correlating patterns with function. Unfortunately, the technique fell into disuse by radiologists while still in early stages of development, and was abandoned by engineering companies when commercial development became uncertain and improvements became costly.

Early thermography as with traditional radiographic mammography depends on vision for interpretation. As with any visual technique, the critical eye of the interpreter is a factor in accuracy and reproducability. As thermology has improved and developed better and more detailed imaging techniques, scanners, and digital data storage capacity, the ability to develop reliable thermography is more assured. The early liquid crystal and infrared techniques have been replaced by high-resolution cameras that can scan more than 10 frames per second, and by very fast focal plane array cameras able to record more than 100 frames per second. Dynamic area telethermometry (DAT) equipment can produce thermal images with a precision of 0.001 degree Celsius. This allows one to detect skin temperature changes produced by normal hemodynamics during the cardiac cycle. Now that's fine tuning! DAT data collection may vary from a few seconds to a few minutes and may utilize from 256 to 1024 consecutive images for analysis.[23] By this technique one can assess a small cancerous lesion's effect on blood-flow dynamics in a substantial portion of the breast.

Because thermology is without risk, one method to increase sensitivity is to obtain serial images over time, thus increasing the accuracy of diagnosis while avoiding the radiation hazard associated with traditional mammography.

French researchers have developed a 24-hour thermographic technique to monitor breast temperature changes, much as a patient with heart problems can be evaluated with a 24-hour heart monitor. The technique is based upon evidence that breast surface temperature reflects tissue metabolism; that there is a relationship between tumor growth rate and thermal and vascular reactions; that the early appearance of thermovascular disorders are associated with breast malignancy "even at the in situ or microinvasive stage"; and that the finding of "alteration of the circadian rhythm of skin temperature is observed in animal and human breast cancers, even at the early stage of tumor growth."[24] This latter finding is very important and may be a clue to not only the physiology of growing tumor cells, but to alterations in hormonal status *preceding* the development of malignancy.

A temperature change in a breast lesion can be caused by any one or a combination of three mechanisms: increased metabolism; increased blood flow as may be found in an abnormal growth; and/or thermoregulatory dilation or constriction of blood vessels. A woman's normal breast is about 5 degrees Celsius lower than her core body temperature. Furthermore, a normal breast develops vasoconstriction when cooled; thus, cooling prior to a thermographic evaluation can be used to accentuate an abnormality.[25]

Dr. Michael Anbar, thermology expert from the University of Buffalo, has suggested that nonneurological vasodilation of cancerous breast tissue is modulated by nitric oxide.[26] Nitric oxide has been shown to be produced by cancerous cells, and its level in the breast may be enhanced by iron-containing ferritin that occurs in greater concentration in cancerous tissue.[27] This abnormal production of nitric oxide appears to be a local reaction, producing changes in blood flow in a cancerous breast, resulting in a pattern different from that of the other breast. This may explain the observed differences in circadian rhythm reported earlier.[28,29] Subtle changes in modulation of breast perfusion due to the presence of cancerous cells may be detected by dynamic area telethermography, the thermal difference resulting from nitric oxide vasodilation or increased blood flow.[30,31]

Still another technique, seldom mentioned in the United States, is the "electronic bra." The procedure, called Electrical Impedance Tomography, or EIT, uses a specially designed brassiere to detect tiny changes in electrical current as it passes through a womans' breast. The bra is connected to an ordinary computer, and the level and pattern of current within the cells produces an image to detect areas of abnormality.[32]

If ever there was a needed alternative to x-ray mammography, thermology seems to be it. Data so far indicate that dynamic thermography has the potential to surpass traditional and static-point-in-time mammography in the study of and diagnosis of breast malignancy. With the exception of ongoing studies at a few centers, questions abound why this harmless, non-invasive, and less costly technique of diagnosis and study has essentially been abandoned in the United States. Although the technique is used in Japan, Austria, and Germany, Dr. Anbar thought three factors were blocking development of thermography in the United States: (1) lack of funding for research from the National Institutes of Health, (2) opposition from established radiology, and (3) reluctance of the insurance industry to pay for such examinations.[33] The insurance industry has an additional incentive not to accept thermography. The technique was utilized for awhile to document soft tissue injury following industrial or other injures; thus, it tipped the balance of proof away from the insurance industry to the patient. A safe, noninvasive, inexpensive, and reliable method of breast surveillance is more than ever a necessity. We must ask, if Congressional and industrial leaders in the United States can invest millions in the technology of heat-seeking missiles, how long will it be before they are willing to invest at least as much money, time, and expertise in heat-seeking techniques to diagnose and study breast cancer? I think women deserve a straight answer.

In summary, each of these techniques, traditional mammography and thermography, is diagnostic only. We must never lose sight of the fact that *early detection* is just that, a way to find a cancer; it does absolutely nothing to *prevent* a cancer from developing.

REFERENCES

1. Both documents are available from the Medical Board of California, 1426 Howe Avenue, Suite 54, Sacramento, CA 95825. FAX: 916-263-2479
2. Gofman, J. W., O'Connor, E. X-rays: Health Effects of Common Exams. Sierra Club Books, San Francisco, CA. pp. 217–227, 1985.
3. Gofman, O'Connor. Op. cit., p. 227.
4. Gofman, J. W. Preventing Breast Cancer: The Story of a Major, Proven, Preventable Cause of This Disease. Committee for Nuclear Responsibility, Inc. PO Box 421993, San Francisco, CA 94142. 1996.
   This table was adapted by Dr. Gofman from his book, pp. 172–181.
5. Bertell, R. Breast cancer and mammography. Mothering. 49–57, Summer, 1992.
6. Gofman. Op. cit., p. 353.
7. Webster, E. W. In: Everyday Radiation. Rosenthal, E., Ed. Sci. Digest, p. 96, March 1984.
8. Segal, M. Mammography facilities must meet quality standards. FDA Consumer. FDA Pub. No. 94-8284, March 1994.

9. Rovner, S. Standards set for mammograms. Washington Post. Health. p. 18. November 15, 1994.

10. Mintz, J. Clinton announces new mammogram rules. Washington Post. p. A-7. October 26, 1997.

11. A. M. A. Medical News. p. 18. April 12, 1976.

12. Bailar, J. C. III, Gornick, H. L. Cancer Undefeated. New Engl. J. Med. 336(22): 1569–1574, 1997.

13. Segal. Op. cit.

14. Elmore, J. G., Barton, M. B., Moceri, V. M., Polk, S., Arena, P. J., Fletcher, S. W. Ten-year risk of false positive screening mammograms and clinical breast examinations. New Engl. J. Med. 338(16): 1089–1096, 1998.

15. Gladwell, M. How safe are your breasts? New Republic. 22–28, October 24, 1994.

16. Blume, S. S. Social process and the assessment of a new imaging technique. Internat. J. Technol. Assess. Health Care. 9(3): 335–345, 1993.

17. Isard, H. J., Sweitzer, C. J., Edelstein, G. R. Breast thermography: A prognostic indicator for breast cancer survival. Cancer 62(3): 484–488, 1988.

18. Anbar, M. Quantitative dynamic telethermometry. Medical Diagnosis and Treatment. CRC Press, Inc., Boca Raton, FL. p. 85. 1994.

19. Elliott, R., Wang, F., Head, J. Relationship of abnormal thermogram to risk of breast cancer and it's prognostic value. American Academy of Thermology. Scientific Program, April 30, 1994.

20. Usuki, H. Computerized analysis of breast thermography and histological findings in breast cancer. American Academy of Thermology. Scientific Program. April 30, 1994.

21. Lilienfeld, A. M., Barnes, J. M., Barnes, H. I. An evaluation of thermography in the detection of breast cancer: a cooperative pilot study. Cancer 24: 1206–1211, 1969.

22. Beahrs, O. H., Shapiro, S., Smart, C., McDivitt, R. W. Supplemental and Concluding Report of the Working Group to Review the NCI/ACS Breast Cancer Detection Demonstration Projects. J. Nat. Cancer Inst. 62(3): 699–707, 1979.

23. Anbar, M. From phenomenological thermography to pathophysiologically based thermal imaging—Twenty five years of clinical thermology. IEE EMBS Magazine 17: (4): 25–33, 1998.

24. Gautherie, M., Yahyai, A., Dehlinger, S., De Prins, J., Walter, J. P. Computerized chronothermodynamic breast examinations under ambulatory conditions. Chronobiol. Int. 7(30): 239–243, 1990.

25. Cary, J., Kalisher, L., Sadowsky, N., Mikkie, B. Thermal evaluation of breast disease using local cooling. Radiology. 115: 73–77, 1975.

26. Anbar, M. Hyperthermia of the cancerous breast: analysis of mechanism. Cancer Lett. 84: 23–29, 1994.

27. Thomsen, L. L., Niles, D. W., Happerfield, L., Bobrow, L. G., Knowles, R. G. Nitric acid synthase activity in human breast cancer. Brit. J. Cancer. 72(5):

41–44, 1995.

28. Wilson, D. W., Phillips, M. J., Holliday, H. W., Blamey, R. W. Prolactin and breast skin temperature rhythms in postmenopausal women with primary breast
cancer. Chronobiologia. 10: 21–30, 1983.

29. Gautherie, M., Yahyai, A., Dehlinger, S., DePrins, J., Walter, J. P. Computerized chronothermodynamic breast examinations under ambulatory conditions. Chronobiol. Int. 7: 239–243, 1990.

30. Anbar, M. Mechanism of hyperthermia of the cancerous breast. Biomed. Thermol. 15(7): 135–139, 1995.

31. Anbar, M., Breast cancer. In: Quantitative Dynamic Telethermometry in Medical Diagnosis and Management. CRC Press, Inc., Boca Raton, FL. pp. 83–94, 1994.

32. Anon. Financial Times of London. p. 8. July 16, 1998.

33. Telephone interview with Dr. Anbar, 12-5-97.

5

RADIATION
FROM BIKINI ISLAND TO LONG ISLAND

I call Heaven and Earth to witness this day: I have put before you
life and death, blessing and curse.
Choose life—that you and your offspring shall live.
—The Bible, Deut. 30:19

RADIATION UNKNOWN

Recently I gave a seminar to a group of about 100 students, science majors at Millersville University in Pennsylvania, and asked for a show of hands from those who had not heard about Three Mile Island (TMI). To my surprise, more than a few raised their hands. When TMI released its radiation on February 28, 1979, many of the students had not yet been born, so perhaps not knowing is somewhat understandable. On the other hand, it is difficult to comprehend this lack of information. The university is situated in Lancaster County, an easy bicycle ride from the TMI power plant, situated on a small island in the Susquehanna River.

Does this deficit in knowledge result from lack of curiosity, from lack of education, or is it a head-in-the-sand reaction to an ongoing source of hazard? Whatever the reason, what we do not know and what we do not pay attention to may, in the end, cause us harm.

For this reason, it is necessary to have some perspective on the history of radiation exposure. Except for cosmic radiation, and that which emanates from certain rock formations, radiation hazards are a new man-made phenomenon, threatening life for fewer than seven decades.

RADIATION FORGOTTEN

The short-term memory of this nation appears remarkably impaired: a kind of collective Alzheimer's condition . . . whether this impairment is purposeful or by neglect remains to be seen.

A slim volume, *Operation Crossroads—The Official Pictorial Record,*[1] of the first atomic bomb tests on the Marshall Islands, published over 50 years ago, is enough to give a person nightmares. How did these tests and subsequent releases of radioactive material from 800-plus bomb detonations remain so buried in the public's memory?

In a foreword to the book, Vice Admiral Blandy, the Commander of Operation Crossroads, wrote of the atomic bomb: [it] "is the most lethal destructive agent yet devised by man. Its energy release is staggering; its radioactivity is slow-killing poison."

Prior to the blasts ·on Bikini Atoll, three atomic bombs had been detonated, the first on July 16, 1945, in the desert near Alamogordo, New Mexico, and the next two, less than a month later, over the Japanese cities of Hiroshima and Nagasaki. Despite evidence of overwhelming death and destruction, the official opinion was that the bombs dropped on the cities in Japan "were of little significance from a technical point of view. They did provide data concerning the effect of the bomb on a city of the Japanese type; but this [sic] data was entirely in the form of rough estimates, proving little."[2] Amazing is the power of language.

Witnessing the two Bikini tests were 42,000 persons, all male except for 37 women nurses. Cameras, which recorded more than 50,000 stills and 1,500,000 feet of movie film, revealed details that the human eye could not tolerate. Among the observers were members of all the military services, civilian scientists, and politicians. One photograph memorializes five Congressmen dressed in business attire and parachutes at Washington's National Airport preparing for their trip to the Pacific test site.[3]

Bikini is a tiny island, sitting upon a coral cap thousands of feet thick. Part of the Marshall group of islands, Bikini is situated 2000 miles southwest of Hawaii. It has a lagoon some 20 miles long and half as wide. Bikini is 250 miles north of Kwajalein, the base for *Dave's Dream,* the B-29 that carried the bomb. The Bikini lagoon afforded anchorage for a range of ships to be tested by both aboveground and undersea detonations. The first blast, named Test Able, occurred on July 1, 1946. The second, the more destructive underwater blast, named Test Baker, was released on July 25th, 9:00 AM Bikini time.

This was an exercise in killing: "The islands were sprayed with DDT to insure healthful condition of the Task Force personnel,"[4] and "Rotenone [a pesticide toxic to fish] was placed in the current along the outer reef, and fish gathered in as they came to the surface," so that they might be identified and tested.[5] Bikini had been an idyllic tropic island connected to others of the atoll by shallow submerged reefs, affording a plentiful supply of fish. The tepid 82 degree F water was perfect for swimming, but swimming was "banned immediately after Test Able until the extent of radioactivity contamination could be determined. Contamination proved negligible and the ban was lifted."[6] Today the atoll is advertised as a scuba diver's paradise. A Bikini dive master said "everybody who likes wreck diving is dying to go there."[7] So much for a reality check.

For the bomb tests, sailors were lined up on the decks of ships, their backs to the blast origin, shielding their eyes with their arms.[8] The rising column of vapor, steam, spray, smoke, and radioactive fission products fed the mushroom cloud, "the radioactivity of which was roughly equivalent to what would exist in the vicinity of 100 tons of radium."[9] As this cloud "spew[ed] forth its insidious content into higher altitudes"[10] the lagoon was deemed "safe," largely by Geiger-counting methods, and personnel entered the area the same day as the blast.

Despite being heavily contaminated and labeled "Danger! Very Radioactive," the target submarine *Skate* was put back into operation by her crew a few days after Test Able.[11] Sailors "washed" other craft with fire hoses prior to reboarding. Divers, wearing shorts and scuba gear, were sent below to photograph the bomb's effects: "The lagoon was found to be covered with many feet of fine silt, pulverized coral resulting from the bomb's explosive force. . . . Divers sank into this silt up to their shoulders. Jagged coral heads and radioactivity added to the difficulties."[12]

"The Test Able shot has been described as a 'self-cleansing' shot since the bomb was detonated in the air and the upward column of gases served to remove most of the radioactive fission products from the lower atmosphere." Lest we derive comfort from the knowledge of widespread dispersion of radioactive materials over the world, the quote continues: "This 'cleansing action' was not experienced to the same extent in Test Baker, in which the bomb was detonated underwater."[13]

Plants were studied for possible radiation-induced mutations, and some fish specimens, obtained before and after the blasts, were sent to Washington, D.C. for study. "The National Cancer Institute supplied white mice with predilections for or against cancer. They were exposed in order to determine whether the intense radiations would produce genetic changes. The mice were returned to the Institute immediately after Test Able to be bred and studied."[14] Many animals were exposed on Bikini, including pigs, goats, rats, mice, guinea pigs, and humans.

For Test Baker, the bomb was detonated underwater. The bomb produced a radioactive cloud fully 2200 feet in diameter, formed from 10 million tons of water hurled into the air. The blast produced intense gamma and neutron bombardment, making radioactive the water's iodine, potassium, and sodium, and produced greater casualties to the test animals than the Able bomb. Gravitation took over and the intensely radioactive water fell to earth. The expanding cloud of spray and water produced radioactivity in the lagoon that "persisted for weeks."[15] The water flowed in and out of the lagoon with the tides, mixing with the ocean currents. Meanwhile the remaining radioactive cloud drifted off with the winds.

When the test ships returned to West Coast ports, radioactive residue was found in saltwater lines and condensers of vessels from the Crossroads tests. What illnesses were to develop in the Navy personnel and shipyard workers exposed to radioactive isotopes and the ever-present asbestos have not been calculated.

One of the last photos in the aforementioned book is of a goat, suffering from radiation sickness. Fifteen percent of the exposed animals died from effects of radioactivity. Incredibly, it is written: "No exact parallel can be drawn between these figures and estimates of the possible effect of the bomb upon human life."

It was against this background that, 6 years later, with my Bachelor's degree earned, I went to work as a radiation monitor at the "Rad Lab"—the Radiation Laboratory—run by the Atomic Energy Commission (AEC) on the University of California campus in Berkeley. It was a new experience to fill out a security clearance form, and though I entered "human" where it asked for race, I received a clearance to work.

To start, I was given a stack of books, at least 8 inches high, and told to read them cover to cover to learn about radiation. My college majors had been in biology and chemistry, so radiation physics and biology was a new and interesting subject, an interest I have maintained through the years.

As a radiation monitor, it was my job to check various laboratories and processes for escaping radiation. I carried with me a Geiger counter, and a more specialized alpha-counter, and on some occasions wore a respirator and protective gloves. These were heady days at the Rad Lab with separation of plutonium having been achieved, operation of the cyclotron, discovery of several of the transuranic isotopes, and characterization of a number of radioactive isotopes. It was at Berkeley where Dr. John Gofman discovered two isotopes of uranium and two more of the rare element protactinium, and where Dr. Melvin Calvin did his elegant work unraveling the process of photosynthesis.

In addition to pure science research, cancer patients were treated through the University/AEC program. I recall a number of patients with polycythemia rubra vera, a malignancy of the red cells, being treated with radioactive phosphorus (P 32) which concentrated in the person's bone marrow. On one occasion I monitored an operating room at a nearby hospital as radioactive gold was instilled into a woman's abdomen to treat her ovarian cancer. My Geiger counter needle was off the scale as I was standing near the doorway. I have no idea whether any of those treatments helped the patients.

The idea that radioisotopes localized in tissues and caused damage became apparent to me when I monitored some of the astatine experiments. The total amount of astatine in the earth's crust totals less than 1 ounce.[17] Astatine occurs naturally in uranium ore, but it is one of the rarest elements in nature because it is one of the most unstable: half of any given amount produced decays in only 8.5 hours. Scientists artificially created the short-lived astatine in the laboratory by bombarding bismuth with alpha particles, accelerated to great speeds in the university's cyclotron. Astatine belongs to the same halide chemical family as fluorine, chlorine, bromine, and iodine, and like iodine, astatine concentrates in the thyroid gland. In addition to concentrating in the thyroid, astatine produced mammary and pituitary tumors after a single injection. Following the work at the University of California, identification and measurement of elementary reactions of astatine have been accomplished at Brookhaven National Laboratory.[18]

This phenomenon of localization and action was a revelation to me, and has served me throughout my scientific life. By knowing the chemical family of an element, one could, with reasonable certainty, predict its site of action and its effect upon living matter.

I accepted an opportunity to work directly in biological research and so transferred to the Navy Radiation Defense Laboratory, situated at the Hunter's Point Naval Shipyard in San Francisco. It was there that we subjected hundreds and hundreds of rats to the effects of thermal and radiation burns. When I left the laboratory in 1954, there was absolutely no doubt in my mind that radiation was harmful, producing effects proportional to exposure.

Despite what had been learned from the research and the enormity of destruction from the Crossroads nuclear blasts, these were not to be the last. One hundred and four nuclear devices were detonated by the United States in the Pacific area. There were 21 additional tests on Bikini, 43 on Enewetok, 12 on Johnson Atoll, and 24 on Christmas Island. Between 1945 and 1989, there were 831 bomb tests. The first were conducted in the atmosphere, and after 1962, mostly belowground in the United States. Of these, 814 were exploded at the Nevada Test Site. Other test sites for underground explosions were Carlsbad, New Mexico; Grand Valley, Colorado; Rifle, Colorado; Farmington, New Mexico; Central, Nevada; Fallon, Nevada; Bombing Range, Nevada; two at Hattiesberg, Mississippi; and three at Amchitka, Alaska.[19] The last United States nuclear test occurred in Nevada in 1992.

And what became of the Marshall Islanders? The Bikini population, numbering 161 persons, was removed from their island home to Rongerik, a mere 130 miles to the east. Rongerik, one-sixth the size of their homeland, had inadequate water and food, and within a few months, the Bikinians were near starvation. They were evacuated first to Kwajalein, then to Kili Island, also lacking a lagoon the people required for fishing.

On March 1, 1954, Bravo, the first hydrogen bomb, was detonated on the surface of Bikini reef. This blast, 1000 times more powerful than the preceding bombs, sent radioactive debris more than 20 miles into the air, drifting over naval ships stationed 40 miles away and over Marshallese on inhabited islands. Citizens on Rongelap and men aboard the Japanese fishing vessel *Lucky Dragon* developed signs of radiation sickness and one died; while on Bikini, radiation levels increased.

In the early 1970s three extended families returned to Bikini until reevacuated in September 1978, when their of water and food supply was deemed contaminated with strontium 90 and cesium 137. Of greater concern, plutonium 239 and 240 were measured in the urine of islanders. Plutonium, with a half-life of 24,360 years, is absorbed by the bone marrow, where it releases harmful alpha radiation as it decays. Commenting on the islanders, Robert Conrad of Brookhaven National Laboratory said the findings "are probably not radiologically significant."[20] In 1954, the fallout from a hydrogen bomb test released on Bikini Atoll reached nearby Rongelap. Examinations by Dr. Rosalie Bertell found that of 76 "unexposed" Marshall Islanders who returned to Rongelap in 1957, 60% had lowered blood monocyte counnts as f 1961. By 1982–86, only 13.7% of 58 remaining Rongelapese had entirely normal blood counts. As for the population who were exposed to the radioactive fallout, as of 1993, Brookhaven National Laboratory with U.S. Congressional funding, still had not released complete blood count data on the exposed Rongelapese.[21]

RADIATION REMEMBERED

This speculation brings us a half century later and halfway around the globe from Bikini Island to Long Island. There are questions about Long Island's Brookhaven National Laboratory (BNL) and other nearby nuclear facilities' contributions to cancer in adults and children. New York States' Attorney General charged that BNL's owner, Associated Universities, "had covered up evidence of widespread contamination, quoting an expert who described it as 'an unanalyzed, undocumented nuclear waste dump.'"[22]

The release of radioactive materials into the air and water by BNL and the surrounding nuclear power plants, combined with widespread chemical contamination, are suspected to be significant factors in the breast cancer epidemic among the people living in Nassau and Suffolk counties of Long Island. A $19 million study to address the issue of high breast cancer rates on Long Island barely addresses chemical pollution—and the radiation issue, not at all.

A look at any map showing either cancer incidence or cancer deaths demonstrates that no cancers are randomly distributed throughout the population—not any cancers, not anywhere in the world, not even lung cancer.

Assuming that the smoking habit is fairly evenly distributed across the United States population, we find that lung cancer is not randomly distributed, and has changed in distribution over time. Analysis indicates that the pattern of lung cancer is due to factors in addition to smoking cigarettes. Radiation damage may compound the natural and synthetic chemical components of cigarettes. Radiation fallout adheres to plants and to tobacco leaves, which have a stickiness about them. Phosphate fertilizer contains uranium and uranium decay products. Alpha-emitting polonium 210 is in the sticky tars of tobacco and stays in the lungs, typically in one spot for 10 days.[23] Thus, together, the radioactive isotopes and nonradioactive chemicals are inhaled in the stream of smoke.

Breast cancer, like every other cancer, is not randomly distributed in the population. It is for this reason that study of Long Island and its epidemic of breast and other cancers is so important. At a public meeting on Long Island, held at East Hampton's Guild Hall on December 5, 1997, it was revealed that the New York State Cancer Registry data showed shockingly high breast and prostate cancer incidence rates in eastern Suffolk County for the years 1989–1993, for which it could offer no explanation.

This new information was compared with the data that had been published in Dr. Jay M. Gould's book *The Enemy Within*.[24] The previously released New York State Cancer Registry data showed age-adjusted breast cancer incidence rates for 62 community groupings for the period 1978–87 in which the combined rate for five towns located on the southern perimeter of BNL was 124 cases per 100,000 women. This was 30% higher than the Suffolk County average of 95 cases. Learning this in 1997, residents of the towns of Brookhaven, Bellport, Yaphank, Shirley, and Medford filed a $1 billion lawsuit against BNL after admission that groundwater flows from the lab had contaminated private drinking-water wells in their area.

Earlier, in the summer of 1997, Dr. Helen Caldicott and Dr. Jay M. Gould, in an op-ed piece published in *Suffolk Life*, reported that the New York State Health Department (NY-SHD) had refused to release cancer data for the 62 community groupings for the years 1989–93, although the department had reported a significant increase of 16% for breast cancer for Suffolk County over the previous 1978–87 period. The more recent age-adjusted breast cancer incidence rate for Suffolk County was 110 cases per 100,000 women, as against the previously reported 95 cases per 100,000.

Under pressure from a Suffolk County Legislative Task Force that was considering the effects of Brookhaven discharges, the NY-SHD offered to give the task force the updated cancer incidence rates for the following three zones of Suffolk County: a central zone consisting of all towns within 15 miles of BNL, a western zone of all towns west of the central zone, and an eastern zone consisting of towns east of the central zone. Considering both breast and prostate cancer, the western and central zones had age-adjusted rates for 1989–93 that were not significantly different from the county

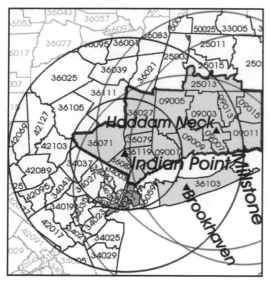

Millstone 1, 2, & 3
Initial criticalities 10/26/70, 1/17/75, and 1/23/86
Located 3.2 miles west-southwest of New London, CT

Haddam Neck
Initial criticality 7/24/67
Located 9.5 miles southeast of Middletown, CT

Brookhaven
Started in 1950
Located in central Suffok County, NY

Indian Point 1, 2, & 3
Initial criticality 8/2/62, 5/22/73, and 4/6/76
Located 3 miles south of Peekskill, NY

Figure 5.1
Map of the Long Island area showing Haddam Neck, Millstone, Indian Point, and Brookhaven reactors. Source: *The Enemy Within,* Gould, J., p. 236. Used with permission of the publisher, Four Walls, Eight Windows, New York.

average, but for the east zone, which included the affluent North and South Folk regions of the Peconic River, the rates were far too high to be attributed to chance. For breast cancer, the East End age-adjusted rate had risen by 72% from 75 to 129 cases per 100,000, and was 17% above the county average. The prostate cancer incidence was also significantly higher than the county average.

At the December 5th meeting in East Hampton, statistician Dr. Jay M. Gould pointed out that had the updated rate for the contaminated five towns south of BNL registered the 16% increase in age-adjusted breast cancer incidence attributed to the county, it would currently be about 143 cases per 100,000 women, possibly the highest single area rate in New York State.

If the high rate of 129 cases per 100,000 women in the East End is found to be centered in the area of the North Fork of the Peconic River, then several factors may be in operation. Situated only 15 miles away from the North Fork are the Millstone reactors, located on the Connecticut shore of Long Island Sound. Wind-borne radioactive discharges from the Millstone plant may share with BNL the responsibility for the East End cancer epidemic. Liquid discharges from BNL, contaminated with radioactive tritium

Millstone 1, 2, & 3, Haddam Neck, Brookhaven, and Indian Point 1, 2, &3

Cumulated per capita emissions of radioactive iodine and strontium from these reactors since 1970s are five times the national average. There are eight counties closest to the four reactor sites. They have a current age-adjusted combined breast cancer mortality rate of 31 deaths per 100,000—the highest in the nation—as well as significantly greater than average increases since 1950–54. Note, too, the high combined rate for the 29 counties within 100 miles of these reactors.

Millstone 1, 2, & 3, Haddam Neck, Brookhaven, and Indian Point 1, 2 & 3

White Female Breast Cancer Mortality Rates 1950–89
Counties within 50 and 100 Miles of Millstone,
Haddam Neck, Brookhaven, and Indian Point

Deaths per 100,000 Women

County	ST	Age-Adjusted Mortality Rates			Percent Change		Number of Deaths		
		1950–54	80–84	85–89	80–84/ 50–54	85–89/ 50–54	50–54	80–84	85–89
Indian Point									
Westchester	NY	30.7	30.7	32.0	0%	4%	586	943	1011
Orange	NY	26.4	29.6	28.3	12%	7%	133	219	238
Rockland	NY	24.3	29.9	33.1	23%	30%	69	220	265
Putnam	NY	38.9	36.1	27.7	-7%	-29%	29	76	67
Dutchess	NY	20.5	26.2	26.6	28%	30%	95	201	222
Above 5 Counties		28.3	30.1	30.7**	6%	8%	912	1800	1883
Brookhaven									
Suffolk	NY	23.2	31.3	32.4**	35%	40%	232	1140	1285
Haddam Neck/Millstone									
Middlesex	CT	22.7	23.7	24.7	4%	9%	49	107	119
New London	CT	22.4	26.8	28.2	20%	26%	97	197	223
2 Counties		22.5	25.6	26.8**	14%	19%**	146	304	342
Total 40 Counties		30.1	29.3	28.8**	-3%	-4%	15015	21466	21859
Total New York City		31.8	29.4	28.3**	-8%	-11%**	6817	6102	5755
Total United States		24.4	24.9	24.6	2%	1%	91392	167803	178868

**P<.001

Figure 5.2
Breast cancer rates in the area surrounding the Haddam Neck, Millstone, Brookhaven, and Indian Point Reactors. Source: *The Enemy Within*, Gould, J., p. 236, used with permission of the publisher, Four Walls, Eight Windows, New York, NY

and strontium 90 have entered the Peconic River, which divides the east end of Long Island into the North and South Fork areas.

Mary Joan Shea, a Long Island cancer activist, knowledgeable in radiation issues, wrote: "Most of the population on Long Island is within a fifty-mile radius of the BNL (Brookhaven National Laboratory), the Shoreham reactor and the Millstone reactors in Connecticut. If you include a 100-mile radius, Long Island women are exposed to at least eight nuclear reactors—Millstone 1, 2, and 3 in Connecticut, Haddam Neck in Middletown, Connecticut, and Indian Point 1, 2, and 3 near Peekskill, New York."[25] It was the Shoreham nuclear plant that resulted in a $5 billion dollar legacy, leading to the nation's highest electricity rates in the nation (Figures 5.1 and 5.2).

Long Island breast cancer activists have urged inclusion of radiation issues[26] in the National Cancer Institute's Long Island Breast Cancer Study Project and submitted several requests to have the water supply tested for radioactive pollutants.[27] They listed at least 13 known Long Island sites as sources of radiation release. Prime among these is BNL, designated a super-fund site because of both radioactive and chemical emissions. "Contaminants have entered the groundwater and plumes have been detected on-site, moving towards the site boundaries, off-site and moving down to the aquifer that is the sole source of drinking water for local communities."[28] These contaminants include radionuclides of uranium, plutonium, cesium 137, cesium 134, strontium 90, tritium, cobalt 60, radium 226, as well as the volatile organic compounds tetrachloroethylene and 1,1,1-trichloroethane.

Long Island has a *sole-source aquifer*. This means that all the water used by people living on Long Island lies, as in a pocket, under the land where they live, work, dump chemicals, apply pesticides, operate incinerators and nuclear facilities, and carry on the various activities of their lives. Rainfall carries the contaminants into an aquifer to mix and migrate throughout the water supply underlying the land. Other communities with sole-source aquifers and the problems of water contamination and cancer are Cape Cod and the islands of Hawaii.

The East End of Long Island includes the affluent Hamptons, whose concerned residents, led by the film actor Alec Baldwin, have established a new environmental organization called STAR (Standing for Truth About Radiation) vehemently oppose wasting federal funds on cancer studies that ignore radioactive contamination of communities. Alec Baldwin's mother, Carol, a Long Island breast cancer survivor, is also engaged in raising funds for objective studies of the causes of cancer in the area.

STAR and the Radiation and Public Health Project (RPHP) are engaged in raising private funds to test levels of strontium 90 (Sr 90) in baby teeth, not only in Suffolk County, but across the entire United States. Germane to the Long Island cancer epidemic are publications by Dr. Gould on the issue of radioactivity and cancer. Included in the *Radiation and Public Health Project* series are "Why cancer rates are highest near New York metropolitan reactors," "Radioactivity levels and cancer in Long Island," and "Radioactive strontium in Long Island baby teeth."[29]

It is this last publication that explains the collecting of baby teeth from across the United States to assay for the radioactive strontium load of young children. Strontium 90, like calcium, is absorbed by bone and teeth. Sr 90 has a half-life of 28 years. A pregnant woman absorbs Sr 90 from her drinking water and diet; consequently, her children's teeth absorb the Sr 90. When children shed their teeth, usually between the ages of 6 and 13, any Sr 90 found in their teeth is an indicator of radionuclides absorbed during intrauterine and newborn life.

Understanding that radioactive chemicals, as first recognized by Rachel Carson, interact with pesticides and other industrial chemicals to cause cancer, STAR and the RPHP hope to replicate the success of the first baby teeth study conducted 40 years ago. This earlier study was led by biologist, ecologist, and educator Dr. Barry Commoner[30] and covered the period of exposure from 1957 to 1961. Dentists in St. Louis, Missouri, collected some 60,000 baby teeth that showed a 20-fold increase in the Sr 90 content of teeth of children born during the peak years of aboveground bomb testing. These findings led to the signing by President Kennedy of the Partial Test Ban in 1963, which ended aboveground bomb testing in the United States.

Since 1992, the German branch of the International Program for the Prevention of Nuclear War, corecipients of the Nobel peace prize, have analyzed 5000 baby teeth. They found a 10-fold increase in strontium 90 in children born in 1986–87, attributable to fallout from the Chernobyl release in the Spring of 1986.

Testing baby teeth for Sr 90 is a simple, inexpensive, noninvasive, and objective way to obtain necessary clinical evidence to coordinate with epidemiological data showing the risk for cancer associated with point sources of ionizing radiation.

Any parent, teacher, physician, dentist, or person interested in public health who wants to contribute children's teeth to the "Tooth Fairy" research study can do so by calling 1-800-582-3716. You will be given instructions on how to send the teeth. Other information on the project is available on the internet as www.radiation.org.

As of January 1999, the measures of Sr 90 in baby teeth are being conducted by radiochemist Dr. Hari Sharma in Ontario, Canada, at the rate of 80 teeth per month. As of February 1999, early results already show that the teeth of children born in Suffolk county zip codes display an anomalous rise from well below one picocurie per gram of calcium for children born in 1977 to levels as high as 8 picocuries per gram of calcium in 1992.

This is already the same rise found in the teeth of children born between 1951 and 1963 that persuaded Kennedy and Khruschshev to terminate aboveground nuclear bomb tests in 1963. The Suffolk County results clearly could not be the result of past bomb tests. RPHP expects to have several hundred teeth analyzed by the Fall of 1999, and will at that time convene a public press conference to announce their results and to point out that the United States is the only one of two dozen nations that has never measured strontium 90 levels in children, and that the RPHP study proves that such studies should continue in order to pinpoint the particular reactor sources of such dangerously high Sr 90 levels. Long Island is not only in proximity to the Millstone, Haddam Neck, Indian Point, and Brookhaven National Laboratory reactors, but is directly downwind from the troubled Oyster Creek reactor, located in Ocean County, New Jersey.

RPHP is hoping to secure foundation support to extend the "Tooth Fairy" project to other areas that have significantly elevated cancer rates.

Given accumulated knowledge about radiation emission hazards, and the unique conditions on Long Island, one must ask why the problem of radionuclide contamination is not included in the Long Island breast cancer epidemic study. Radionuclides are relatively easy to measure, are independent of any patient's memory, and are, unfortunately, stable in the environment and in the body. Radiation emissions, combined with the load of toxic chemicals used and released on Long Island, presents a ticking time bomb.

Antinuclear activist Dr. Helen Caldicott, a pediatrician and former head of Physicians for Social Responsibility, has called for closure and cleanup of the Brookhaven facility. Some parents have expressed concern that rare forms of cancer in their children may be due to releases from the BNL. BNL scientists have formed Friends of Brookhaven to protest suggestions of hazard from operation of the facility, and have labeled as "overreaction" the resident's concerns.

Former Senator D'Amato, a major factor in getting funding for the LIBCSP, when asked about closing BNL said, "I would fight it every step of the way."[31] Still, he did call for closure of the High Beam Reactor at BNL. These issues often boil down to the politics of jobs. Which will result in greater harm—closing BNL to prevent more pollution to the citizens and the environment, or keeping the lab open to preserve jobs. But which jobs? If the spread of radiative pollution continues, there will be a shift in the job market to nurses, chemotherapy and radiation technicians, and bereavement specialists. Which kinds of jobs do we want to support?

Why have we not taken action since Rachel Carson wrote *Silent Spring,* making the connection between radiation, chemical contamination, cancer, and genetic damage? Linked over miles and decades are the Bikini Islanders and the Long Islanders, whose individual suffering could have been prevented.

REFERENCES

1. The Office of the Historian Joint Task Force One. Operation Crossroads—The Official Pictorial Record. Wm. H. Wise & Co., Inc., New York. 224 pages. 1946.
2. Ibid., p. 8.
3. Ibid., p. 45.
4. Ibid., p. 9.
5. Ibid., p. 35.
6. Ibid., p. 71.
7. World Wide Web: Marshall Islands.
8. The Office of the Historian Joint Task Force One. Op. cit., p. 125.
9. Ibid., p. 145.
10. Ibid., p. 141.
11. Ibid., p. 159.
12. Ibid., p. 219.
13. Ibid., p. 143.
14. Ibid., p. 108.
15. Ibid., p. 205.
16. Ibid., p. 220.
17. Weast, R. C., Astle, M. J., Eds. CRC Handbook of Chemistry and Physics. CRC Press, Boca Raton, FL. page B-7, 1981.
18. Weast. Op. cit.

19. Robbins, A., Makhijani, A., Yih, K. Radioactive Heaven and Earth—The Health and Environmental Effects of Nuclear Weapons Testing In, On, and Above the Earth. Apex Press. New York. p. 51. 1991.
20. Niedenthal, J. Bikini Atoll. World Wide Web. 1997.
21. Bertell, R. Internal bone seeking radionuclides and monocyte counts. Internat. Perspect. Public Health 9: 21–26, 1993.
22. Rabinovitz, J. Charges of nuclear cover-up alarm plant's neighbors. New York Times. p. B-7. September 18, 1997.
23. Bertell, R. Personal communication.
24. Gould, J. M. The Enemy Within—The High Cost of Living Near Nuclear Reactors. Four Walls, Eight Windows, New York, London. 1996.
25. Shea, M. J. Letter to R. Allen, Ph.D., National Cancer Institute, Re: Brookhaven National Laboratory and radionuclides. 4 pages. April 22, 1997.
26. Goodman, M. Breast cancer on Long Island: The nuclear connection. Suffolk Life Newspapers. April 4, 1997.
27. Goodman, M. Letter to Gammon, M. D. and Neugut, A. I. September 30, 1996.
28. Shea. Op. cit.
29. Available for a nominal sum ($2.00) from: Radiation and Public Health Project, 302 West 86th Street, Suite 11-B, New York, NY, 10024.
30. Commoner, B. The Closing Circle—Nature, Man and Technology. Alfred A. Knopf, New York. pp. 51–57, 199–200. 1972.
31. Pleven, L. New pressure on lab: Critics mobilize for fight. Newsday. pp. A-1, A-3. October 18, 1997.

6

RADIATION
NUCLEAR AND X-RAY

Concern for man himself and his fate must always be the chief interest of
all technical endeavors . . . in order that the creations of our mind shall be a
blessing and not a curse to mankind. Never forget this in the midst of your
diagrams and equations.
—Albert Einstein,
From an address at the California Institute of Technology, 1931

During the summer of 1997, the media released a story that bombs exploded
at the Nevada nuclear test site between 1951 and 1958 exposed some 160
million people across 3701 counties of the 48 contiguous U.S. states to radiation fallout. Because of radiation carried on air currents and precipitated with
rain, people living in Albany, N.Y., parts of Massachusetts, Missouri,
Tennessee, North and South Dakota, Idaho, and Montana received as much
radiation as residents directly downwind from the Nevada blasts.[1] The
National Cancer Institute (NCI) estimated that the I 131 fallout from the
bomb tests could result in between 11,000 and 212,000 thyroid cancers. Put
into more humane terms, that means that between 11,000 and 212,000 people
could develop thyroid cancer. Mind you, the estimate of effects from bomb
testing considered only I 131 releases and thyroid cancer, not any of the other
isotopes that can cause cancer.

Two panels convened by the National Academy of Sciences analyzed the
NCI data and came to the conclusion there was no need to screen for thyroid
cancer. Rather they proposed to wait for a malignant growth to become
evident, saying there was no evidence of improved survival. Dr. Robert S.
Lawrence, a physician from Johns Hopkins School of Public Health heading

one of the panels, concluded that "a general screening program was not jus-
tified and that it might very well cause more harm than good."[2] The
reasoning was that many thyroid lumps that a physician might feel during a
physical examination are not cancer, and would have to be investigated
further with tissue biopsies.

When a spokesman from the American Cancer Society was asked to
comment on the findings, Dr. Clark Health said "I would not be greatly concerned," and further stated "there's a lot of uncertainty about how one
translates this kind of dose information into actual risk."[3]

If the ACS and the Institute of Medicine from the National Academy of
Sciences are not concerned and are unable to make public health recommendations, who should be concerned, given the mountains of information
generated since the dawn of the atomic age? How can this news be so easily
dismissed?

There is no measurable threshold below which a carcinogenic agent does
not cause harm, as demonstrated in a unique study. Animals were given a
known carcinogen at various dose levels. Those receiving low doses of a
cancer-causing agent developed malignancies, as did those receiving higher
doses, but it took a longer period of time for the cancers to be evident in the
low-dose range.[4]

Early changes in a cell's control machinery are difficult to impossible to
measure. Over time, left unchecked, the carcinogenic changes initiated in a cell
become manifest. Every exposure carries some risk, and multiple exposures
from multiple sources carry more risk, often additive, multiplicative, or
synergistic.

Looking at information to date, we have come to the realization that the
body is assaulted in multiple ways: pollutants from pesticides and other
industrial products; chemical pollutants from incinerators and dumps;
radioactive pollutants from bomb testing, power plant operations, uranium
mines, and leaking disposal sites; each with the ability to act and interact.
Thus, there is little wonder that the breast cancer rate (indeed, cancer of
multiple sites) has increased dramatically over the past four decades. It is
not just that women are living longer, or that there are better diagnostic
methods, the breast cancer rate has risen in each age group. In these four
decades there has occurred the rise of significant technologies: chemical
production, radiation technology, and the "disposal" of each. Breast cancer
is not a coincidence.

Radioactivity is an energy form, exposure to which sets in motion, imperceptibly, events to reveal themselves years to decades later. Each and every incremental exposure to any form of nuclear radiation increases the risk of cancer. It is persistent, deadly, silent, and unseen.

Radiant energy comes in several forms. The commonest and best-known form of man-made radiation energy is that discovered by Roentgen: x-rays, useful in medicine and industry. X-rays are employed to diagnose and treat disease in human and veterinary medicine. X-rays examine our luggage prior to boarding an airplane. X-rays are used in industry and metallurgy, as for example, to determine if pipeline welding seams are secure. Other forms of external radiation are those delivered by the atomic bombs to the people living in Hiroshima and Nagasaki and to the atomic veterans, both military and civilian, exposed in the course of atomic bomb construction and testing.

There are cumulative hazards associated with exposure to low-level amounts of radiation, whatever the source. The type of radiation determines the biological mechanism and damage. For example, penetrating x-ray emissions cease when the emitting source is turned off, and the deadly gamma radiation from a bomb is of short duration. This is not so with other sources of radiation, such as the radioactive isotopes emitted from weapons testing and nuclear power plants. These latter sources, actually chemicals, emit alpha, beta, and gamma forms of ionizing radiation.

Alpha radiation is a charged particle, from the core of an atom, consisting of two protons and two neutrons; beta radiation consists of high-speed electrons escaping from the nucleus of an atom; and gamma radiation is a photon form of energy.

The biological effects of exposure to high-level and low-level radiation are very similar to the consequences of exposure to high and low levels of chemicals. Exposures to each, high enough to kill a cell, may impair body functions. If sufficiently high, radiation exposure may kill. Chronic low-level exposures to either radiation or chemicals may *damage* cells, resulting in impairment of immunity, cell division, hormonal function, and repair mechanisms. It is low-level exposure to both *external* and *internal* radiation that represents risk for the development of cancer.

Gamma radiation emitted by unshielded sources can be of great danger. In Taiwan, around 1983, more than 100 buildings were constructed with steel rods contaminated with the gamma emitter cobalt 60. The source of the radiation was not discovered until 1992. By then, some 6000 citizens had been exposed in residential and school buildings. Taiwanese researchers reported that persons chronically exposed to the low-level gamma radiation developed significantly more abnormalities in the nucleus of their white cells than did two control populations.[5] What this means for their long-term health is unknown at this time. Fortunately, 95% were relocated, an action not taken for the Chernobyl population, as we will subsequently learn.

Internal radiation occurs when radioactive chemicals gain entry to the body, ingested or inhaled. Nuclear power plants and nuclear bombs release all three kinds of radiation: alpha, beta, and gamma. Alpha radiation is especially dangerous because of high energy release from particles as they decay. When these long-lived particles accumulate in tissues, cells are damaged and sometimes killed.[6] The resultant genetic damage to a cell that survives alpha radiation may be transmitted to its progeny many cell divisions later.[7]

The half-life of a radioactive element is a factor in predicting harm. Half-life refers to the time for half a given quantity of an element to "decay" into a lower energy form. Importantly, the new form is not necessarily a less harmful form. With each decay transformation, energy is released, causing damage to cells or tissues, wherever the isotope is located.

To give some scope to the enormity of radiation decay, consider the isotope uranium 238. It has a half-life of 4.5 billion years and undergoes both alpha and beta decay, transforming sequentially into isotopes of thorium, radium, radon, polonium, and bismuth before reaching a stable state as lead. During the decay process, U 238 and its decay isotopes become deposited in various parts of the body, including the bones, kidneys, gastrointestinal tract, and lungs.

The poisonous isotope radium, discovered to cause cancer in women who painted the glow-in-the-dark instruments of World War II, persists for a half-life of 1600 years, appearing but a mere flash when compared to bone-soluble, plutonium 239, with a half-life of 24,390 years. In the history of our earth, plutonium was the primordial isotope. Life did not evolve until most of the plutonium had decayed to uranium.[8]

Uranium, isolated from pitchblende, a rock rich in radioactive elements, was the starting material for isolating plutonium. Beginning in 1944, plutonium was produced artificially from uranium in the first nuclear reactors, ending up in bombs and power plants. Now, the United States has on hand 50 tons of "surplus" plutonium, a powerful alpha emitter that deposits in bone. The Department of Energy proposes to "contain" part of the plutonium surplus in a glass/ceramic vitrification process and to burn the rest in commercial power reactors.[9] The communities where these processes will be carried out will be showered with this most toxic of all chemicals. It appears the citizens are largely unaware, even though the pattern of contamination is predictable, measurable, and most importantly, knowable.

Nuclear half-life and biological half-life, while interrelated in effect, are not the same. Nuclear half-life is characteristic of each individual isotope of an element. The biological half-life is the time span over which the element is resident within a body. Some chemicals are released quickly from the body, excreted in the breath, feces, urine, or breast milk. Still others, such as isotopes of strontium and radium, become embedded in our bones and remain there for years. The radiation released in the process of decay, its path of decay, and the form(s) into which an element decays all have a bearing on effects within the body.

The level of danger from any radioactive material depends on the type of radiation it emits, the amount of energy involved, the half-life of the element, and the biological pathway(s).[10] Radiation operates at various energy states. Gamma radiation, like x-rays, can penetrate solid barriers, including the human body. Alpha and beta forms of radiation penetrate tissue less easily and cause harm in other ways. Alpha particles have the shortest range, but the largest mass, while beta rays, which are high-energy moving electrons, can travel though thousands of cells before being stopped. Radiation forms do damage all along their path of travel. Changes occur in the electrical state of an atom as electrons are knocked out of their former orbits around the nucleus of an element and thus release ionizing radiation. When ionization occurs in a tissue it results in disruption of chemical bonds and of cellular components. Such disruption of normal molecules may result in alteration of an enzyme or protein, mutation of a cellular reproductive function, damage to DNA, or death of tissue. Further discourse on the physics of ionizing radiation are beyond the scope of this book; however, the contribution of radiation to breast cancer and resultant public health ramifications will be discussed.

Radiation is used in the treatment of some malignancies, to kill cancerous cells intentionally. The radiation may be delivered by any one of the energy forms: x-ray, gamma, beta, or alpha radiation, depending upon the site and the needed effect. While the use of medical radiation has undoubtedly prolonged and saved the lives of many, it is not an unmixed blessing. It is the overuse, inappropriate use, and misapplication of this technology that is of concern.

There is no controversy about the contribution of radiation to development of lung cancer,[11] leukemia, and thyroid cancer. Women who were given x-irradiation to follow the course of tuberculosis treatment; for evaluation and treatment of scoliosis; and radiated for treatment of acne, have an increased incidence of breast cancer.[12,13]

X-ray "treatments" were foisted upon women for seemingly benign and self-limiting conditions. Breast radiation and drug administration have been prescribed to "treat" postpartum breast swelling, an admittedly painful but not life-threatening condition that is better controlled with cold packs and a tight-fitting brassiere. A dose-related increase in incidence of breast cancer was seen in women given x-ray therapy for postpartum mastitis, resulting in an increased overall cancer relative risk of 2.2.[14] Similar findings of increased breast cancer in women radiated for benign breast disease were reported from Sweden as well,[15] and confirmed by Dr. John Gofman in his extensive analyses.[16] These and similar extrapolations led to the mistaken assumption that there was a linear relation for all forms of radiation exposure.

Dr. John Gofman relates a number of examples of medicine gone awry, where common sense, and maybe even economics, succumbed to the siren song of technology. Eight hundred and fifty patients, 750 of them younger than 7 years of age, were subjected to x-rays to treat whooping cough at the Boston Floating Hospital in the 1920s.[17] At the Mayo Clinic, more than 1000 patients were given x-ray treatment of asthma.[18] Considering the comprehensive records maintained by the Mayo Clinic, it would be of scientific value to know who, among the radiated patients, developed breast cancer. At the same facility, countless more patients, with dermatological conditions, were given either x-ray or radium therapy.

Increased cancer risk as a result of early-age radiation exposure led Dr. Gofman to express concern for sick neonates, often radiated multiple times to diagnose and correct life-threatening abnormalities and conditions.[19] There is no question as to the trade-offs; early death versus later risk, but a reason to limit radiation to procedures of absolute necessity. Even "routine" chest or dental x-rays carry some risk of cancer. It is the unneeded forms of x-ray we must avoid, keeping in mind that radiation procedures have saved lives.

Addressing breast cancer specifically, Dr. Gofman's research shows that when a woman receives significant radiation prior to the age of 20, she is more likely to develop breast cancer before the age of 35. Japanese women, exposed to the atom bombs at ages as young as 10 years, experienced a greater incidence of breast cancer than those similarly exposed at age 35 or older, suggesting "the breast tissues of adolescent females may be more sensitive than those of older women to the effects of ionizing radiation."[20] Mouse offspring, subjected to gamma radiation in utero, when followed through their lifetime, displayed not only leukemia, but mammary cancer as well.[21] This may explain why "Baby Boomers" are experiencing a higher rate of breast cancer different from previous rates for women of this age group who were born before bomb testing and nuclear power reactors released their isotopes into the biosphere.[22]

Twenty-five years ago, Dr. Gofman and his associates outlined their observations concerning the effects of radiation, reiterated in 1981 and still true. Essentially they are:

- All forms of cancer can be induced by radiation, all having similar increases with increased radiation exposure.
- It takes less radiation at young ages to increase cancer mortality than for adults.
- The cancer rate per radiation unit is reached earlier with predominantly alpha emissions.[23–25]

The early findings of Dr. Gofman and his associates were not without hazard to themselves; they were attacked by the nuclear establishment, threatened with cuts in both funding and staff.[26]

Capturing the conflict between the development of technology and hazards to society, the author Catherine Caufield wrote: "At the heart of the debate were two very different hazards to society—the hazard of disease and genetic damage and the hazard of totalitarianism."[27] There is concern that neither hazard has decreased to a safe level in our time.

The International Physicians for the Prevention of Nuclear War (IPPNW), corecipient of the 1995 Nobel prize for peace, have published an easily understood compendium of when, where, and how radiation was released worldwide by nuclear testing, and details how poor has been control of emissions.

To describe in words the adverse effects of radiation is not an easy matter. One can begin with Carole Gallagher's *American Ground Zero—The Secret Nuclear War*.[28] Ms. Gallagher's interviews with and photographs of citizens living primarily in Utah and Nevada, close to our nation's atomic weapons test site, are stark and graphic. One person, Augusta Peters, with a soft smile that matches her curly hair, stares straight into the camera. One notices that her chest caves in as a result of double mastectomies. If *they,* who made decisions to explode those nuclear bombs, receive her stare, would they dismiss her story of radiation exposure as one of the calculated costs of nuclear preparedness?

Cost: a useful and interesting word that has had a metamorphosis. A document uncovered by Ms. Gallagher, in the cost-benefit context, offers a frightening example of the failure of ethics and morality. An Atomic Energy Commission (AEC) memo describes the people living downwind from the Nevada test site as "a low use segment of the population."[29]

Those "downwinders" might well ask who benefited from being a member of "a low use segment of the population"? If it was not the radiation-exposed citizens, who was it, and how did it come about? Let us explore.

A pattern of ignorance and denial emerges when one reads accounts of Gallagher's radiation victims and survivors. Denial is a common personal defense when one is confronted with an intolerable situation, impossible to change, but ignorance is inexcusable. Ignorance results from two forces: absence or misleading information and/or refusal to learn. In the downwind area from the Nevada test site, all factors were in operation: misinformation, lack of information, unwillingness to look at what was available, and of course, denial. It is not simply denial by the affected population, but by government as well. It is denial that must be combatted.

While those living in Nevada and Utah bore the brunt of the bomb releases, radioactive fallout spread eastward. Radiation's adverse effects were well known before the bombs were set off in the desert dawn. The adverse effects became more and more apparent with each blast. Complaints of human illness and harm to livestock exposed to fallout were reported, were "investigated," and were suppressed.[30] Extensive research was carried out on animals exposed to radiation's effects. This author worked on such a project in 1953 at the Navy's Radiological Defense Laboratory in San Francisco. Even then, with but a Bachelor's degree, I understood the harmful effects of nuclear radiation. And I was not alone.

It shouldn't have required four decades to make a decision to put public health ahead of nuclear destruction, but until Department of Energy Secretary Hazel O'Leary came into office, it did not appear to be a high priority with either the Atomic Energy Commission (AEC) or its successor, the Nuclear

Regulatory Commission (NRC). And neither, it appears, has the National Cancer Institute (NCI) considered radiation-induced cancer of high priority, taking 15 years to release its report.

The Nevada bomb-test site is not the only source of radioactive pollution. Uranium was mined, milled, purified, and fashioned not only into bombs, but put into power-generating facilities, and as we learned from the Gulf War, into munitions. Tailings, the leftover rock from mining, was used for fill and road construction, spreading contamination across the landscape.

Radioactive materials are handled, transported, used, and stored throughout this country, indeed all over the world. Adding to the radioactive load is contamination carried by the winds from the Soviet Union's tests, the Chernobyl catastrophe,[31] and bomb tests undertaken by the United States, France, Britain, China, India, Pakistan, and others. Radiation that contaminates a community need not come from nearby. The intense radiation measured in 1953 in Albany, New York, came from a bomb test at the Nevada Test Site, the fallout cloud passing 40,000 feet overhead, and carried to earth in a thunderstorm.[32,33]

Comparing breast cancer incidence in 1967–75 with a 1951 cohort, Dr. Carl Johnson found a near doubling of breast cancer in Utah women who lived in the fallout path from the Nevada test site. He found 27 cases versus 14 expected cases.[34] Radiation-induced breast cancer susceptibility is increased when exposure occurs in adolescence and early adulthood,[35] and is promoted by hormonal stimulation.[36] Japanese atomic bomb survivors have increased breast cancer.[37,38]

The catastrophic effect of nuclear bombs leads any thinking person to support their ban, but ignored are releases from nuclear power plants, which for the most part, and with a few stunning exceptions, run quietly, out of sight and out of mind. Even when releases became public as from Three Mile Island in Pennsylvania, the Fermi plant in Michigan, the Sellafield facility in Britain, and Chernobyl in the Ukraine, there is practically no public outcry, and the events are wiped from conscious memory.

It is not that these hazards came unannounced. The hazards from nuclear radiation were heralded worldwide by independent researchers: Dr. John Gofman,[39] Dr. Carl Johnson,[40,41] Dr. Thomas Mancuso,[42] and Dr. Ernest Sternglass[43] in the United States; Dr. Alice Stewart[44] in Britain; Dr. Rosalie Bertell[45] in Canada; and Nobel laureate Andrei Sakarov[46] in the Soviet Union, all of whom warned of widespread adverse effects.

The enormous costs to build and maintain nuclear power plants is leading to closure of plants and storage of their accumulated radioactive materials, posing yet another set of perils. Underground storage is proposed, but the earth is subject to earthquakes, floods, storms, migration of materials, and terrorism. We have no idea if this technology will actually contain these long-lived toxins or not. Unappreciated by the public are the enormous costs, not only of construction, but of transport, containment, and security. And security may prove to be the most elusive of all.

A clear demonstration of a slow learning curve is the current push to build nuclear reactors in China. In this effort, Westinghouse Electric Corporation, Asea Brown Boveri, Inc., and Bechtel Corporation have joined in a lobbying and public relations effort to stress domestic jobs.[47] The reasons that no new United States nuclear plants have been ordered since 1973 seems to have escaped the public. Do we not understand that radioactive emissions know no boundaries?

A common emission from the nuclear industry, radioactive strontium (Sr 90), becomes deposited in bone with a half-life of 28 years. Sr 90 decays by the release of powerful beta radiation, which damages the bone marrow, the site of blood cell and immune cell formation. In terms of power, the beta radiation of Sr 90 travels relatively long distances, creating free-radical (ionization) changes as it passes through a large volume of tissue. This ionization initiates physiologic and biochemical changes in cells within the bone marrow.[48]

More than 50 years ago, an issue of the *Journal of the American Medical Association* described delayed effects upon immune competency and blood formation in men and women exposed at Hiroshima.[49] Adverse effects upon immune function from Sr 90 were confirmed in the 1970s by Sternglass and by Ito and colleagues.[50,51] Dr. Rosalie Bertell studied four separate populations, all of whom had been exposed to bone-seeking radionuclides. These affected people spanned the globe: a Toronto suburb; Bukit Merah, Malaysia; Rongelap in the Marshall Islands; and the Mississauga First Nation living on the north shore of Lake Huron. She found lowered monocyte counts in all four groups.[52] Monocytes are formed in the bone marrow and are required in sufficient numbers to fight infection and provide immune function.

Data supporting adverse effects upon immune function are those of Gould and Sternglass, who found an excess of between 20,000 and 40,000 deaths during the summer of 1986. Those disproportionally affected were the elderly and those with infectious diseases, and coincided with the areas in the United States that received the greatest fallout from Chernobyl.[53] We know little of the effects upon the Lapland Finns and their reindeer herds who were the first to recognize the spread of contamination from the Chernobyl explosion. Infant mortality and stillbirths rose in areas of Germany receiving the greatest Chernobyl fallout,[54] but by far, people living in the vicinity of the plant were harmed the most. The Chernobyl residents have a marked increase in cancer, immunological abnormalities, birth defects in their children, and even more ominous, permanent genetic damage. Of some 32,000 "liquidators," mostly men between the ages of 35 and 45, who worked on the containment after the Chernobyl explosion, more than 32,000 have become invalids, and some 8000 have died. The testimony of victims, scientists, and observers of the terrible consequences of nuclear power is detailed in *Chernobyl: Environmental, Health and Human Rights Implications.*[55]

Compounding fallout from the Chernobyl release was a United States hydrogen bomb test, called Mighty Oaks, that went badly wrong in April of the same year.[56] The Department of Energy test blast released radioactivity from the test shaft into the atmosphere, and fallout was measured as far away as Burlington, Ontario.[57]

There is no way of knowing exactly how much of the current cancer epidemic is related to nuclear bomb production and testing since the 1940s, and from the current operation of nuclear power reactors. There has been no concerted program to document and map radiation releases from all these sources, but given the known hazards and persistence of radiological isotopes, there is significant reason for concern.

An isotope of specific concern for breast cancer is cesium (Cs 137), which is released from nuclear power and bomb production facilities. Cs 137 emits beta particles, with a half-life of 30 years. Cs 137 is in the same family of chemicals as sodium and potassium. Common to sodium and potassium, Cs 137 and its isotopes concentrate in soft tissues, including breast, liver, spleen, and muscle, resulting in near total body radiation during the decay period.

As for strontium (Sr 90), the adverse effects upon the bone marrow are not the only concern. As Sr 90 decays it transforms into yttrium 90 (Y 90), which concentrates in glandular organs, including the pituitary gland. The pituitary, located deep within the brain, is the "master gland" that controls

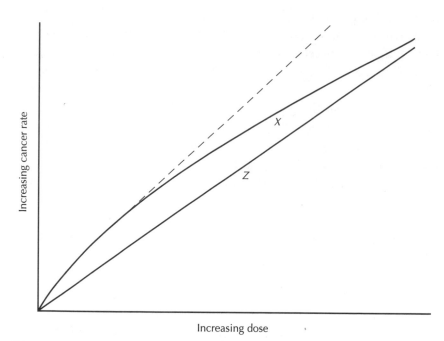

Figure 6.1
Supralinearity: Increasing cancer rate and increasing dose.

the endocrine system.[58] Various hormones released from the pituitary gland control function of the ovaries and testes, adrenal and thyroid glands, and growth hormone and prolactin secretion. Prolactin is the stimulant that causes breast cells to produce milk.

Very low levels of radiation exposure have been demonstrated to cause an enhanced, supralinear effect due to free-radical release, resulting in functional and physiologic effects, not necessarily due to genetic or mutational damage. Supralinearity, as shown in Figure 6.1, simply means that there is an enhanced effect at low doses. Curve Z demonstrates a linear, straight-line relationship between dose and effect. Curve X demonstrates supralinearity, that is, a greater effect or response at low doses compared to higher ones. If the lower part of curve X were extended outward over the range of doses, as shown by the dotted line, the adverse effects would be greater than actually measured.

This sort of low-level damage includes changes in red cell permeability and membrane integrity, that is, the ability of substances to leak in and out of cells. It involves susceptibility to infection, and changes in antibody response and antibody production.[59-61] Low-level effects from radiation are echoed in similarly enhanced effects from chronic, low-level exposure to such chemicals as dioxin,[62] and in the adverse effects upon the behavior and the reproductive organs of animals exposed to very low levels of bisphenol-A and other estrogenic chemicals.[63]

In other words, one must not become lulled into complacency because doses are low. Exposure to low doses over time, and to doses of multiple agents, either chemical and radiological, or both, carries a measure of harm.

Epidemiology, the least sensitive of techniques employed to assess connections between exposure and risk, has demonstrated a link between proximity to radiation-emitting facilities and breast cancer. Adding to the epidemiological data are human case reports, animal experiments, and biological research. Ordinarily, with this much concurrent proof of cause and effect, one should expect performance to protect the publics' health. Unfortunately, this has not been customary.

A case in point are the findings of Drs. Thomas Mancuso and Alice Stewart, two pioneers in the field of radiation hazards, whose 1977 publication demonstrated a link between radiation exposure and death from cancer in the Hanford nuclear workers. These researchers found:

- Radiation levels were always higher for deaths from cancer as compared to noncancer deaths.

- The cancer/noncancer ratio contrasts were greater for deaths after 50 years of age than for deaths of younger persons.

- In three age groups, the proportion of cancer deaths was highest for those receiving the top cumulative radiation dose.[64]

Linking disability data with death certificates, Dr. Mancuso found cancer greatly underreported, with breast cancer deaths among women employed at the Hanford facility not reported 60% of the time.[65] This is a serious omission, since when death data are underreported, a suspected risk becomes hidden and a source of hazard is not addressed.

The same year, Dr. Carl Johnson, director of health for Jefferson County, Colorado, echoed Mancuso's link between radiation exposure and cancer, and reported increased leukemia in persons living near the Rocky Flats plutonium processing facility, located outside of Denver.[66,67] Rocky Flats was a nuclear weapons plant whose plutonium and other radionuclide exhaust releases date from 1953.[68] Dr. Johnson compared cancer rates in the population living closest to the Rocky Flats facility with those in more distant suburban areas and found that by 1969–1971 there was a 15% overall excess cancer incidence. Those closer to the facility had malignancies that included leukemia, lymphoma, myeloma, and cancers of the lung, thyroid, breast, esophagus, stomach, and colon.[69]

Dr. Mancuso's study of the Hanford radiation workers was one of the longest running ever undertaken, involving 35,000 employees, and initially funded by the AEC. When an excess of cancer deaths among the workers was also reported by Washington epidemiologist Dr. Milham in 1974, the response of the AEC was to put pressure on Dr. Mancuso to refute Milham's finding. This, Dr. Mancuso could not do. The next year, the AEC phased out Dr. Mancuso's contract and transferred the study to an in-house group, based at Oak Ridge. In light of the current industry demands for "peer review" these events are all the more revealing, brought out in hearings before a House of Representatives Subcommittee, chaired by Paul Rogers: "It was disclosed at the hearings that the transfer of the project to Oak Ridge had not been preceded by a request for proposal, that there was no peer review of the contractors, no research protocol, and no principal investigator."[70] One is left with the impression that the decision to stop Dr. Mancuso's research was based not upon science, but upon political and economic factors. While Dr. Mancuso's study of Hanford workers was stopped, the radiation emissions have not stopped. In a 1996 survey of Oregon women living downwind of the Hanford area, researchers found a high rate of hypothyroidism and associated spontaneous abortion,[71] confirming what had been reported *30 years* previously by Dr. Ernest Sternglass.[72]

When Dr. Alice Stewart joined Dr. Mancuso's group, she had retired from Oxford University after a career of 33 years. In the years following, Dr. Stewart argued for a halt to the conflict of interest between the Energy Department's various functions and its assessment of radiation effects. She pointed out that the Energy Department is the owner and operator of nuclear weapons sites; it is the principle repository for data on exposed workers, who have but limited access to their own data; and it is the source of funding for radiation-exposure studies.[73] In other words, it is like asking Dracula to guard the blood bank.

Nearly two decades later, using U.S. Department of Energy (DOE) data, Joseph Mangano found the Oak Ridge National Laboratory in Tennessee had released Sr 90, Cs 137, and I 131 into the local water supply. Released

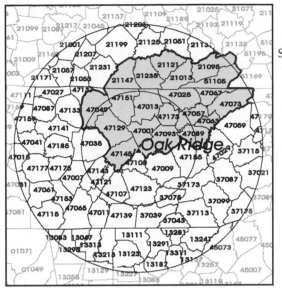

Oak Ridge
National Laboratory
Selected on September 9, 1942,
as a uranium enrichment site.
Code named Site X
In full operation with 80,000
employees by late 1994.
Located 20 miles east of
Knoxville, TN

Figure 6.2
Map of area surrounding Oak Ridge National Laboratory. Source: *The Enemy Within,* Gould, J., p. 252. Used with permission of the publisher, Four Walls, Eight Windows, New York.

also into the air and water were other radionuclides, mostly before 1960. An examination of death records found a 31.8% increase in cancer deaths between the periods 1950–1952 and 1987–1989, continuing to rise from 1988 to 1989, and ahead of the age-adjusted rate of the entire United States. In Anderson County, where the Oak Ridge facility is located, the cancer deaths rose 39.1% compared to a rise of 29.5% in the 12 counties located over 40 miles distant. In the mountainous counties, where rainfall is greater, the cancer mortality was 40.4% compared to 30.3% in the lowland regions. Three downwind counties recorded a cancer death rate increase of 50.8%, compared to a 7.1% increase in four upwind counties.[74]

For comparison, 40 years previously, the cancer mortality in the Oak Ridge area was uniformly below the national average, as demonstrated in Figures 6.2 and 6.3.

Drs. Ernest Sternglass and Jay M. Gould provide compelling evidence linking releases from nuclear power plants and the epidemic of breast cancer on Long Island. The researchers reviewed releases from reactors

"As one of the nations's oldest reactor sites (along with Hanford and Los Alamos), Oak Ridge has contributed to a 38 percent increase in the combined age-adjusted breast cancer rate of a group of 20 down-wind counties. As in the case of all other DOE reactor sites located in rural areas with below-average initial mortality rates, the subsequent mortality increases are too large to be attributed to chance."
—Gould.

Oak Ridge National Laboratory

White Female Breast Cancer Mortality Rates 1950–89
Counties within 50 and 100 Miles of Oak Ridge

Deaths per 100,000 Women

County	ST	Age-Adjusted Mortality Rates			Percent Change		Number of Deaths		
		1950–54	80–84	85–89	80–84/ 50–54	85–89/ 50–54	50–54	80–84	85–89
Anderson	TN	18.7	21.6	23.9	16%	28%	17	50	58
Campbell	TN	14.6	28.8	20.4	97%	40%	9	35	29
Claiborne	TN	21.9	20.9	15.1	-5%	-31%	10	15	12
Fentress	TN	4.1	23.2	6.4	458%	54%	1	10	4
Grainger	TN	20.6	13.9	16.8	-33%	-18%	6	7	9
Hamblen	TN	3.8	17.3	22.7	351%	492%	2	24	39
Hancock	TN	22.3	7.3	44.4	-68%	99%	4	1	9
Hawkins	TN	20.6	22.0	21.7	7%	5%	13	30	30
Jefferson	TN	15.7	21.5	25.3	36%	60%	7	23	28
Knox	TN	19.1	22.8	22.1	19%	16%	95	225	231
Morgan	TN	3.5	12.8	16.4	266%	368%	1	7	9
Roane	TN	21.6	16.9	16.5	-22%	-24%	14	27	30
Scott	TN	10.7	15.1	12.2	40%	14%	3	7	7
Union	TN	10.7	13.1	28.2	22%	162%	2	5	11
Bell	KY	5.1	23.1	21.5	350%	318%	4	24	22
Harlan	KY	11.0	15.8	22.1	43%	100%	11	21	28
Knox	KY	15.3	19.9	27.6	31%	81%	9	18	29
Mc Creary	KY	3.5	17.7	23.3	405%	564%	1	7	10
Whitley	KY	19.3	18.4	21.7	-5%	12%	13	21	25
Lee	VA	6.3	24.2	18.5	284%	194%	4	20	18
Total 29 Counties		15.5	20.8	21.4	34%	38%**	226	577	638
Total 71 Counties		15.8	20.6	20.4	30%	29%**	578	1522	1652
Total United States		24.4	24.9	24.6	2%	1%	91392	167803	178868

**P<.001

Figure 6.3
Breast cancer rated in counties surrounding Oak Ridge National Laboratory.
Source: *The Enemy Within,* Gould, J., p. 253. Used with permission of the publisher, Four Walls, Eight Windows, New York.

located most closely to Long Island and New York City. These included the reactors at Indian Point, which began operation in 1961; the Haddam Neck facility, which started in 1967; and Millstone, which began operation in 1970. The combined releases from these three facilities between 1970 and 1987 "was more than three times the 14.2 curies reported for the Three Mile Island" reactor release of 1979.

Such comparisons are fraught with problems, not the least of which may be arguments of "safety" by proponents of nuclear industry. The Long Island area reactors had releases occurring over some 17 years, while official measurement of the TMI radiation did not begin until the Saturday following the Wednesday morning leak, resulting in underestimation of the full occurrence. For either area, releases were significant.

The Millstone reactor, 10 miles north of Suffolk County in Connecticut, "released 32.6 curies of airborne I 131 and other fission products, and 581 curies of liquid fission products by 1987, most of it in the period 1972–1979." Coincident rises in breast cancer mortality were seen in Nassau and Suffolk

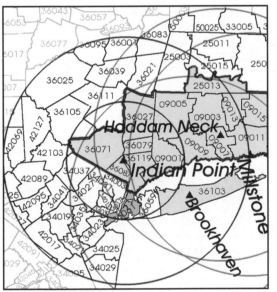

Millstone 1, 2, & 3
Initial criticalities 10/26/70,
1/17/75, and 1/23/86
Located 3.2 miles west-southwest
of New London, CT

Haddam Neck
Initial criticality 7/24/67
Located 9.5 miles southeast
of Middletown, CT

Brookhaven
Started in 1950
Located in central
Suffolk County, NY

Indian Point 1, 2, & 3
Initial criticality 8/2/62, 5/22/73,
and 4/6/76
Located 3 miles south
of Peekskill, NY

Figure 6.4
Map of the Long Island area showing Haddam Neck, Millstone, Brookhaven, and Indian Point Reactors. Source: *The Enemy Within,* Gould, J. Used with permission of the publisher, Four Walls, Eight Windows, New York.

"Cumulated *per capita* emission of radioactive iodine and strontium from these reactors since 1970s are five times the national average. There are eight counties closestto the four reactor sites. They have a current age-adjusted combined breast cancer mortality rate of 31 deaths per 100,000—the highest levels in the nation —as well as significantly greater than average increases since 1950–54. Note, too the highcombined rate for the 29 counties within 100 miles of these reactors."
—Gould.

Millstone 1, 2, & 3, Haddam Neck, Brookhaven, and Indian Point 1, 2 & 3

White Female Breast Cancer Mortality Rates 1950–89
Counties within 50 and 100 Miles of Millstone,
Haddam Neck, Brookhaven, and Indian Point

Deaths per 100,000 Women

County	ST	Age-Adjusted Mortality Rates			Percent Change		Number of Deaths		
					80–84/	85–89/			
		1950–54	80–84	85–89	50–54	50–54	50–54	80–84	85–89
Indian Point									
Westchester	NY	30.7	30.7	32.0	0%	4%	586	943	1011
Orange	NY	26.4	29.6	28.3	12%	7%	133	219	238
Rockland	NY	24.3	29.9	33.1	23%	30%	69	220	265
Putnam	NY	38.9	36.1	27.7	-7%	-29%	29	76	67
Dutchess	NY	20.5	26.2	26.6	28%	30%	95	201	222
Above 5 Counties		28.3	30.1	30.7**	6%	8%	912	1659	1803
Brookhaven									
Suffolk	NY	23.2	31.3	32.4**	35%	40%	232	1140	1285
Haddam Neck/Millstone									
Middlesex	CT	22.7	23.7	24.7	4%	9%	49	107	119
New London	CT	22.4	28.8	26.2	20%	26%	97	197	223
2 Counties		22.5	26.6	25.8**	14%	19%**	146	304	342
Total 40 Counties		30.1	29.3	28.8**	-3%	-4%	15015	21466	21859
Total New York City		31.8	29.4	28.3**	-8%	-11%**	6817	6102	5755
Total United States		24.4	24.9	24.6	2%	1%	91392	167803	178868

**P<.001

Figure 6.5
Breast cancer rates within the area surrounding Haddam Neck, Millstone, Indian Point and Brookhaven reactors. Source: The Enemy Within, Gould, J., p. 237. (Used with permission of the publisher, Four Walls, Eight Windows, New York.

counties on Long Island paralleling the increase in Connecticut, located across Long Island Sound. Peaks in mortality appear to have occurred 7 to 9 years after the startup of the Haddam Neck and Millstone reactors with a 39% increase in deaths in Suffolk County alone for the 3-year periods, 1970–1972 and 1987–1989. It is but ten miles across Long Island Sound from the Millstone reactor to the North Fork of Suffolk County.[75]

Figures 6.4 and 6.5 demonstrate the location of the three reactors and the breast cancer rates in counties downwind from those reactors.

The breast cancer epidemic on Long Island is under study by Columbia University and is funded by the National Cancer Institute. Nuclear radiation is not included as a part of the official NCI research. An independent and parallel research project by Dr. Jay M. Gould and a panel of experts from the Radiation and Public Health Project is conducting a study of the radiation load on the citizens of Long Island.

Dr. Gould has made a call for parents to contribute baby teeth to be tested for radioactive strontium (Sr 90). These teeth, shed when a child is about 6 years of age, are a record of the radioactive material transferred to that child from the time of conception.[76] Dr. Gould hopes the findings may explain why cancer is so high in areas of Long Island that lie in the path of nuclear drift, of both recent and remote release.

The 1990 National Cancer Institute Study "Cancer in Populations Living Near Nuclear Facilities"[77] found no excess cancer in 107 counties in which such facilities were located. Expanding the number of "exposed" counties beyond that used by NCI, Drs. Gould and Sternglass found the contrary. They criticize the NCI for including as "controls" some counties well within the fallout area of about 50 to 100 miles downwind from a reactor. The NCI misclassification increased the "control" baseline against which "nuclear" county death rates were measured, so that no significant difference could be detected.

For white women with breast cancer, Gould and Sternglass found a "significant upward deviation from the national trend . . . in 268 counties within 50 miles of reactor sites." For 53 nuclear reactor sites that started operation before 1982, the average increase was highest, compared with a 1% increase in breast cancer for the United States as a whole. They found the greatest rise in death rates in the counties surrounding the facilities built in the years 1943 to 1953 that released fission products such as I 131 and Sr 90. These included the nuclear facilities at Hanford, Washington; Oak Ridge,

Tennessee; Idaho National Engineering, Idaho; Savannah River, Georgia; Los Alamos, New Mexico; and Brookhaven, New York. All six sites had increased breast cancer deaths for the periods 1950–1954 and 1985–1989, ranging from 11% to 333%, with an average of 33%.[78]

Accompanying the 1990 NCI study that was published in the *Journal of the American Medical Association* was a remarkable statement:

> It is somewhat ironic that public concern over the potential hazards of normally operating nuclear facilities receives much greater attention than the far greater risks imposed by such voluntary life-style factors as smoking, drinking and diet.[79]

In other words, blame the victim. What about the women with breast cancer who did not smoke, did not drink alcoholic beverages, and exercised, but did drink radiation-contaminated water, and did eat dairy products, meat, fruits, vegetables, grains, and oils produced in the fallout zones of bomb tests and nuclear reactors? Is this indeed lifestyle?

Such a statement in a publication of the American Medical Association, a well-funded and powerful pressure group, raises other concerns. One is the admonition of Hippocrates who cautioned: "First do no harm." If physicians are not the patient's advocate, who shall be?

The risks to health from radiation exposure have been studied and documented. Linked as well are risks to democracy from suppression and control of vital information. The books by Dr. Gofman, the articles by Dr. Sternglass, and the recent book by Drs. Gould and Goldman document radiation releases and the adverse effects upon human health and the environment.[80,81] Exposure data support a link between consumption of radioactive contaminated dairy products and cancer. The data do not support the "blame the victim," fat-consuming, "lifestyle" argument.

Radioactive forms of strontium and iodine concentrate in the nonfat part of cow and human breast milk.[82] Isotopes of radon, formed during the decay of uranium, thorium, and plutonium, are readily fat-soluble, where they, along with two beta releasers, release alpha particles.[83]

Citizens of central Wisconsin, with a high breast cancer rate, received radioactive fallout, no matter which way the wind blew, ringed as it is by nuclear reactors.[84] Lending evidence to the issue of radioactive contamination of dairy herds is the finding that, of 16 industrial countries studied, only New Zealand, Australia, Hong Kong, and Israel had declines in breast cancer deaths between 1971 and 1986.[85] None of these four had nuclear reactors;

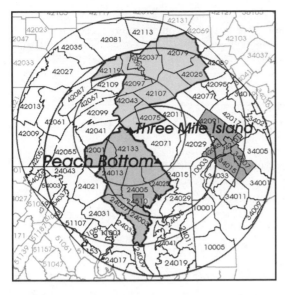

Three Mile Island 1 & 2
Initial criticality 6/5/74
and 3/28/78
Major accident 3/28/79
Located 10 miles southeast of
Harrisburg, PA

Peach Bottom 1, 2, & 3
Initial criticality 9/16/73
and 8/7/74
Unit 1 shut down in 1974
Located 17.9 miles south of
Lancaster, PA

Figure 6.6
Map of Pennsylvania's Three Mile Island and Peach Bottom reactors. Source: *The Enemy Within,* Gould, J., p. 238, Used with permission of the publisher, Four Walls, Eight Windows, New York.

however, the southern hemisphere countries of New Zealand and Australia must have received some contamination from tests conducted by France in the south Pacific, and from the British weapons testing at Monte Bello and Maralinga in Australia. Hong Kong is very near the reactor built by mainland China and also must have received some fallout from Chinese nuclear tests.

Israel is one of the better examples of reducing the confounding factors of nuclear fallout and pesticide pollution. While Israel has an advanced nuclear reactor program, Israeli breast cancer deaths, highest when world-wide fallout was greatest between 1976 and 1986, fell 34%, coinciding with restriction of chlorinated pesticide use and cessation of atmospheric nuclear tests in 1980.[86] While the exact contribution of each risk is still unmeasured, and perhaps unknowable, that should not stop society from limiting exposure to these known hazards.

In five counties adjacent to the Three Mile Island reactor, breast cancer "increased markedly following normal operation after start-up at TMI and following the accident."[87] Reading that quote again, one is stuck not so much by the admission of risk from the accident, but the risk from "normal operation." Critical words in the sentence are "normal operation." We must

"The 16 counties closest to these reactors have registered a significant 13 percent increase in breast cancer mortality since 1950-54. Their combined current rate of 27 deaths per 100,000 is close to the nation's highest. The same could be said for the even higher combined rate for all counties within a radius of 100 miles."
—Gould.

Three Mile Island 1 & 2 and Peach Bottom 1, 2 & 3

White Female Breast Cancer Mortality Rates 1950–89
Counties within 50 and 100 Miles of
Three Mile Island and Peach Bottom

Deaths per 100,000 Women

FIPS Code 85–89	County	ST	Age-Adjusted Mortality Rates			Percent Change 80–84/ 85–89/		Number of Deaths		
			1950–54	80–84	85–89	50–54	50–54	50–54	80–84	85–89
Three Mile Island										
42043	Daupin	PA	24.5	25.4	28.8	3%	17%	141	212	240
42075	Lebanon	PA	22.3	24.5	25.5	10%	14%	50	100	106
42097	Northumberland	PA	25.3	31.4	29.8	24%	18%	83	139	141
42107	Schuylkill	PA	24.8	24.1	28.1	-3%	13%	134	184	199
42119	Union	PA	18.5	14.4	25.5	-22%	38%	12	17	25
42093	Montour	PA	22.5	35.5	25.5	58%	13%	15	26	20
42037	Columbia	PA	19.6	29.7	33.1	51%	69%	31	70	73
42079	Luzerne	PA	22.6	25.2	25.5	11%	13%	243	383	387
42025	Carbon	PA	19.5	20.7	25.3	6%	29%	31	52	67
Total	9 Counties		23.3	25.6	27.2*	10%	17%	740	1183	1258
Peach Bottom										
42071	Lancaster	PA	26.6	27.2	25.2	2%	-5%	182	351	356
42133	York	PA	24.5	27.9	26.1	14%	6%	143	294	309
24013	Carroll	MD	20.7	21.0	25.8	2%	25%	28	58	86
24005	Baltimore	MD	27.5	24.9	28.4	-10%	3%	174	540	650
24025	Harford	MD	13.9	21.3	24.8	54%	79%	14	72	99
24027	Howard	MD	16.3	27.6	27.9	70%	72%	8	66	90
24003	Anne Arundel	MD	22.2	30.1	27.5	35%	24%	44	262	279
Total	7 Counties		24.6	26.2	26.8**	7%	9%*	593	1643	1869
Total	Above 16 Counties		23.9	26.0	27.0**	9%	13%**	1333	2826	3127
Total	56 Counties		26.2	27.0	27.2**	3%	4%	6079	10226	11010
Total	United States		24.4	24.9	24.6	2%	1%	91392	167803	178868

Figure 6.7
Breast cancer rates within the area of Three Mile Island and Peach Bottom reactors. Source: *The Enemy Within,* Gould, J., p. 239. Used with permission of the publisher, Four Walls, Eight Windows, New York.

guard against believing that just because wrong technology has persisted, that it is *normal* or acceptable. A further example must be taken from the civil rights arena: slavery was once a "normal" method of doing business.

Research done by volunteer canvassers, working with Drs. Carl Johnson and Bruce Moholt, determined the cancer rate around Three Mile Island was 7 times that of similar rural areas.[88] Revealed as well were mutations in plants, reminding us that *all* living matter is subject to the laws of nature.

A 1990 Columbia University study found no association between cancer and proximity to releases from the 1979 TMI accident. Once again, faulty assumptions and legal constraints led to underestimation of effects. More recently, analysis of the TMI data by Dr. Wing and his associates found an increase in all cancers, particularly lung cancer and leukemia.[89] The breast cancer rate is graphically presented in Figures 6.6 and 6.7.

But Dr. Wing's study came too late to help the victims. In February 1987, Judge Lipsett, presiding in the case against Metropolitan Edison, the operator of TMI, dismissed the claims of 35 plaintiffs stating:

> At the time of the accident, these plaintiffs were certainly aware of the release of radiation and threatened harm from such a release. . . . They also knew or should have known that exposure to a radiation could cause adverse effects.[90]

In other words, if you "knew or should have known" there was a hazard to your health, you are out of luck. This same defense has been used successfully to quash claims of harm from cigarettes, incinerators, pesticides, and toxin-emitting factories. Considering recent developments in cigarette litigation, perhaps victims can hope for justice from the legal system. Realistically, this closeout maneuver has been used successfully against persons harmed by dangerous industries and dangerous products. Will the emerging political climate allow for redress for injury? We must consider very thoughtfully and carefully our options. They are decreasing in number.

Restricting access to information or redress is not new. Those controlling the nuclear industrial-military complex often cite "national security" as justification to exclude the citizen, whose very life and well-being is at risk. But to be fair, data control is well-established in the corporate world as well, citing "business confidentiality" as an overt reason, while of equal importance are *control and profit.* In many cases, military and nonmilitary nuclear development and corporate control and profit are one. Martin Marietta operated Oak Ridge, Three Mile Island was owned by Metropolitan Edison, and Rocky Flats was operated by Rockwell International Corporation.

The report of the Advisory Committee on Human Radiation Experiments released on October 21, 1994, contains information applicable not only to the issue of breast cancer, but to civil rights as well. The document states: "Experiments involved the *intentional* [emphasis added] environmental releases of radiation that (A) were designed to test human health effects of ionizing radiation; and (B) were designed to test the extent of human exposure to ionizing radiation."[91]

It is unlikely we will ever know the true number, extent, or type of intentional radiation releases, but that document discloses the following, and these are direct quotes:

> Eight radiation warfare experiments; the number is at least 53; Four Los Alamos, New Mexico imploding tests involving radiolanthanum. DOE reports that the number of such tests approximates 250; One intentional release from a plutonium production facility (Green Run). Examples of further releases from nuclear production facilities have been found.[92]

Governmental agencies involved in these intentional exposures included the CIA with its "MKULTRA program of experiments [which] included radiation research; however, as the CIA previously reported, Director of Central Intelligence, ordered MKULTRA files destroyed in 1973," and the Naval Radiological Defense Laboratory (NRDL) which operated from 1947 until "disestablishment in 1969, [when] its library of research reports was evidently dispersed, and basic records were apparently destroyed." The DOE's Intelligence division's "critical data on intentional releases and work done for others . . . revealed that these files were essentially purged during the 1970s and as late as 1989," and "in the 1960s, NASA contracted with DOE's Oak Ridge operations to perform a retrospective study of whole body radiation" [that] encompassed over 3000 radiation exposures at over 40 institutions. . . . In 1981 congressional testimony, NASA stated that the data had been destroyed in the *Routine course of business.*"[93]

Recently declassified documents discuss a United States "'radiological warfare' program 'to release highly radioactive substances by dropping them in bombs' . . . 'in the form of pellets, aerosol or dust [that] would escape and spread,' preserving an industrial base, while destroying its skilled workers." Additional plans included "'large scale sabotage use' in which radioactive gases or aerosols would be injected with germ sprays into natural gas mains,' rendering the victims 'more susceptible to infection from the germs.'[94]"

Senator John Glenn in his opening statement as Chairman of the Hearings before the Senate Committee on Governmental Affairs on Human Subject Radiation said: "It is becoming increasingly clear that all too often the over-riding reasons for the classification of many of the radiation experiments records was not national security, but instead fear of lawsuits and personal culpability." [95]

John Gofman, M.D., Ph.D., world-famous codiscoverer of uranium 233, author of four scholarly books on radiation effects, and Professor Emeritus of Molecular and Cell Biology at the University of California in Berkeley, writes:

> Our surest path toward Orwellian unknowledge in the textbooks is control over the preparation of the input parameters for the databases upon which our knowledge rests. Falsify the database, and the greatest geniuses in the world will arrive at the wrong answer concerning health effects of radiation.[96]

As we come to the end of the 20th century and bomb testing of the 1950s recedes from our consciousness, we recently learn, two months after the fact, that the managers of the Hanford Nuclear Reservation released toxic chemicals mixed with plutonium into the atmosphere. The release was the result of a tank explosion that exposed workers and raised concern as to the fate of the plutonium that remains radioactive with a half-life of 24,360 years. Hanford officials are quoted as saying "they do not believe anyone off-site had any exposure and said the toxic plume appears to have dissipated before it reached the public highway."[97]

Is there anyone who believes otherwise but that *what goes up must come down?* And down where? And where for however many more centuries after the 24-plus centuries to dissipate just half of that release?

The overwhelming accumulation of information leaves little question but that fission products in the diet,[98] acting in concert with chemical pollution, cause harm and result in cancer, birth defects, genetic alterations, and immunological and neurological damage.[99] Repeated exposures and exposures to multiple agents increase risk, often in ways unanticipated. There is little argument but that both chemical toxins and radioactive materials have a compounding effect and increase the dangers of each.

The tragic faces, resulting from the Chernobyl nuclear disaster, mixed with industrial pollution in the former USSR, are evident in deformed children and sick adults graphically portrayed in an issue of National Geographic.[100] How many more of the worlds' people will suffer before we stop nuclear technology?

REFERENCES

1. Associated Press. '50s Nuclear Testing Exposed People Across U.S., Study Says. Washington Post. p. A-15. July 26, 1997.
2. Brown, D. Mass testing opposed for cancer from 1950s fallout. Washington Post. p. A-14, September 2, 1998.
3. Associated Press. Op. cit.
4. Staffa, J. A., Mehlman, M. A., Eds. Innovations in Cancer Risk Assessment (ED 01 Study). J. Environ. Pathol. Toxicol. 3(3): 1–246, 1980.
5. Chang, W. P., Hwang, B-F., Wang, D., Wang, J-D. Cytogenic effect of chronic low-dose, low-dose-rate, gamma radiation in residents of irradiated buildings. Lancet. 350: 330–333, 1997.
6. Johnson, C. J. A cohort study of cancer incidence in Mormon families exposed to nuclear fallout versus an area-based study of cancer deaths in whites in southwestern Utah. Amer. J. Epidemiol. 125(1): 166–168, 1987.
7. Kadhim, M. A., Lorimore, S. A., Hepburn, M. D., Goodhead, D. T., Buckle, V. J., Wright, E. G. Alpha-particle-induced chromosomal instability in human bone marrow cells. Lancet. 344: 987–988, 1994.
8. Bertell, R. Personal communication.
9. Lippman, T. U.S. decides on plutonium disposal plan. Washington Post. pp. 1, 6. December 9, 1996.
10. Graeub, R. The Petkau Effect. Four Walls, Eight Windows, New York. p. 15. 1994.
11. Edling, C., Ed. Lung Cancer and Radon Daughter Exposure in Mines and Dwellings. Department of Occupational Medicine. Linkopong, Sweden. 149 pages. 1983.
12. Boice, J. D., Monson, R. R. X-ray exposure and breast cancer. Amer. J. Epidemiol. 104(3): 349–350, 1976.
13. Simon, N., Silverstone, S. M. Is breast cancer caused by radiation? Int. J. Radiat. Oncol. Biol. Physics. 2(1): 91, 1977.
14. Shore, R., Hemplemann, L., Pasternack, B., Kowaluk, E. Breast cancer following x-ray therapy for acute post-partum mastitis. Amer. J. Epidemiol. 106(3): 230, 1977.
15. Baral, E., Larsson, L., Occurrence of breast carcinoma in women treated with x-rays for benign diseases of the breast in Sweden. Third International Symposium on detection and prevention of cancer. 288–389, 1976.
16. Gofman, J. W. Radiation-Induced Cancer from Low-Dose Exposure: An

Independent Analysis. C. N. R. Books, San Francisco. 1990. (Multiple citations with supporting data.)

17. Bowditch, H. I., Leonard, R. D., Emerson, P. W., Wyman, E. T., Barron, E. W., Green, H., Hubbard, E., Tennis, M. Treatment of pertussis by Roentgen ray. J. Amer. Med. Assoc. 85(3): 171–177, 1925.

18. Leddy, E. T., Maytum, C. K. Roentgen treatment of bronchial asthma. Radiology. 52: 199–203, 1949.

19. Gofman, J. Personal communication. 11-12-94.

20. McGregor, D. H., Land, C. E. Bhoi, K., Tokuoka, S., Liu, P. I. Wakabayashi, T., Beebe, G. W. Breast cancer incidence among atomic bomb survivors, Hiroshima and Nagasaki. J. Nat Cancer Inst. 59(3): 799–811, 1977.

21. Sinja, N., Samuel, K. C., Agarwal, A. Carcinogenic effect of very low doses of antenatal ionizing radiation. Indian J. Cancer. 21: 36–45, 1984.

22. Mangano, J. J. Low-Level Radiation and Immune System Damage: An Atomic Era Legacy. Lewis Publishers, Boca Raton. 1999.

23. Gofman, J. W., Tamplin, A. R. Low dose radiation and cancer. IEEE Transactions on Nuclear Science. Part I. Vol. NS-17, 1-9. February, 1970.

24. Gofman, J. W. Radiation and Human Health: A Comprehensive Investigation of the Evidence Relating Low Level Radiation to Cancer and Other Diseases. Sierra Club Books, San Francisco. 1981.

25. Gofman, J. W., O'Connor, E. X-rays: Health Effects of Common Exams. Sierra Club Books, San Francisco. 1985.

26. Caufield, C. Multiple Exposure. University of Chicago Press, Chicago. pp. 156–158, 1989.

27. Ibid., p. 127.

28. Gallagher, C. American Ground Zero—The Secret Nuclear War. Random House, New York. 360 pp. 1993.

29. Ibid., Prologue. p. xxiii.

30. Smith, R. J. Scientists implicated in atom test deception. Science. 218(4572): 545–547, 1982.

31. Burlakova, E. B., Ed. Consequences of the Chernobyl Catastrophe: Human Health. Center for Russian Environmental Policy, Scientific Council on Radiobiology, Russian Academy of Sciences, Moscow. 249 pp. 1996.

32. Robbins, A., Makhijani, A., Yih, K. Radioactive Heaven and Earth: The Health and Environmental Effects of Nuclear Weapons Testing In, On, and Above the Earth. Apex Press. New York. p. 61. 1991.

33. Sternglass, E. J. Evidence for low-level radiation effects on the human embryo and fetus. Radiation Biology of the Fetal and Juvenile Mammal, Sikoff, M. R., Mahlum, D. D., Eds. Hanford Radiobiology Symposium No. 17. U.S. Atomic Energy Commission. pp. 693–716, 1969.

34. Johnson, C. J. Cancer incidence in an area of radioactive fallout downwind from the Nevada test site. J. Amer. Med. Assoc. 251(2): 230–236, 1984.

35. Bertell, R. Handbook for Estimating Health Effects from Exposure to Ionizing Radiation. Institute of Concern for Public Health, 67 Mowat

Avenue, Suite 343, Toronto, Ontario M6K 3E3, Canada. August 1984. This publication is available in the U.S. from Ministry of Concern for Public Health, 5495 Main Street, Suite 147, Buffalo, NY 14221, as well as in England.

36. Upton, A. C. Biological basis for assessing carcinogenic risks of low-level radiation. Carcinogenesis. 10: 381–401, 1985.

37. Wakabayashi, T., Kato, H., Ikeda, T., Schull, W. J. Incidence of cancer in 1959-1978, Based on the Tumor Registry. Radiation. Res. 93: 112–146, 1983.

38. Tokunaga, M., Land, C. E., Yamamoto, T., Asano, M., Tokuoka, S., Ezaki, H., Nishimori, I. Breast cancer in Japanese A-Bomb survivors. Lancet. October 23, 1982.

39. Gofman, J. W., Tamblin, A. R. Epidemiological studies of carcinogenesis by ionizing radiation. In: Proceedings of the Sixth Berkeley Symposium on Mathematical Statistics and Probability: Effects of Pollution on Health., LeCam, L. M., Neyman, J., Scott, E., Eds. University of California Press, Berkeley, CA. pp. 235–277. 1970.

40. Johnson, C. J. Cancer incidence patterns in the Denver metropolitan area in relation to the Rocky Flats plant. Amer. J. Epidemiol. 126(1): 153–155, 1987.

41. Johnson, C. J. Before Chernobyl: Hanford, Savannah River, and Rocky Flats. J. Amer. Med. Assoc. 257(2): 191, 1987.

42. Holden, C. Low-level radiation: A high-level concern. Science. 204(13): 155–158, 1979.

43. Sternglass, E. J. Environmental radiation and human health. In: Proceedings of the Sixth Berkeley Symposium on Mathematical Statistics and Probability, held in 1971. LeCam, L. M., Neyman, J., Scott, E. L., Eds. University of California Press, Berkeley, CA. pp. 145–216. 1972.

44. Stewart, A. An epidemiologist takes a look at radiation risks. Division of Biological Effects, U.S. Department of Health, Education and Welfare, Public Health Service, Bureau of Radiological Health, Rockville, MD. 88 pp. 1973.

45. Bertell, R. X-ray exposure and premature aging. J. Surg. Oncol. 9: 379–391, 1977.

46. Graeub, R. The Petkau Effect—The Devastating Effect of Nuclear Radiation on Human Health and the Environment. Four Walls, Eight Windows, New York. p. 173. 1994.

47. Morgan, D., Ottaway, D. B. U.S. Reactor firms maneuvering to tap China's vast market. Washington Post. pp. A-1, A-16. October 21, 1997.

48. Petkau, A. Introduction: free radical involvement in physiologic and biochemical processes. Canad. J. Physiol. Pharmacol. 60: 1327–1329, 1982.

49. Keller, P. D. A clinical syndrome following exposure to atom bomb explosions. J. Amer. Med. Assoc. 131: 504–406, 1947.

50. Sternglass, E. J. The role of indirect radiation effects on cell membranes in the immune response. Radiation and the Lymphatic System, Ballou, J. E., Ed. ERDA Symposium Series 37; 185–191, 1976.

51. Ito, T., Nagao, K., Kawamura, Y., Yokoro, K. Studies on the leukemogenic and immunologic effects of radiostrontium (Sr 90) and x-rays in mice. Proceedings of the 14th Annual Hanford Biology Symposium. Ballou, J. E.,

Ed. Technical Information Center Energy Research and Development Administration, pp. 209–217. 1974.

52. Bertell, R. Internal bone seeking radionuclides and monocyte counts. Internat. Perspect. Pub. Health. 9: 21–26, 1993.

53. Gould, J. M., Sternglass, E. J. Low level radiation and mortality. Chemtech. 19: 18–21, 1982.

54. Luning, G., Scheer, J., Schmidt, M., Ziggel, H. Early infant mortality in West Germany before and after Chernobyl. Lancet. 1081–1083, November 4, 1989.

55. Permanent People's Tribunal Session on Chernobyl. Environmental, Health and Human Rights Implications. Vienna, Austria, 12–15 April, 1996. Available from International Medical Commission on Chernobyl, 710-264 Queens Quay West, Toronto, Ontario M5J 1B5, Canada.

56. Caufield, C. Multiple Exposures. University of Chicago Press, Chicago. p. 238. 1989.

57. Bertell, R. Personal communication.

58. Graul, E. H., Hundeshagen, H. Studies of the organ distribution of yttrium 90. Straulen Therapie. 106: 405–457, 1958.

59. Sternglass, E. J. The role of indirect radiation effects on cell membranes in the immune response. In: Ballou, J. E., Ed. Radiation and the Lymphatic System. ERDA Symposium, Series 37, 1976.

60. Petkau, A. Effect of 22Na+ on a phospholipid membrane injury to irradiated human erythrocytes. Radiat. Res. 34: 335–346, 1968.

61. Gofman, Op. cit.

62. Goldstein, J. A., Linko, P., Bergman, H. Induction of porphyria in the rat by chronic versus acute exposure to 2,3,7,8-tetrachlorodibenzo-p-dioxin. Biochem. Pharmacol. 31(8): 1607–1613, 1982.

63. vom Saal, F. S., Cooke, P. S., Buchanan, D. L., Palanza, P., Thayer, K. A., Nagel, S. C., Parmigiani S., Welshons, W. V. The physiologically based approach to the study of Bisphenol-A and other estrogenic chemicals on the size of reproductive organs, daily sperm production and behavior. J. Toxicol. Indust. Health. xx: yy, 1997.

64. Mancuso, T. F., Stewart, A., Kneale, G. Radiation exposures of Hanford workers dying from cancer and other causes. Health Physics. 33(5): 369–384, 1977.

65. Mancuso, T. F. Methodology in industrial health studies: Social Security disability data and the medical care system. Amer. J. Indust. Med. 23: 653–671, 1993.

66. Johnson, C. J. Leukemia death rates of residents of areas contaminated by plutonium. Abstract. Amer. Pub. Health Assoc., Washington, D.C. 11-1-77.

67. Johnson, C. Cancer incidence in an area contaminated with radionulides near a nuclear installation. Ambio. 10: 176–182, 1981.

68. Draft Impact Statement, Rocky Flats Plant Site, 1545-D, United States Energy Research and Development Administration, Golden, CO. 1977.

69. Johnson, C. J. Nuclear Installation Report. Ambio. 10(4): 176–182, 1981.

70. Holden, C. Low-level radiation: a high-level concern. Science. 204: 155–158, 1977.

71. Grossman, C. M., Morton, W. E., Nussbaum, R. H. Hypothyroidism and spontaneous abortions among Hanford, Washington, Downwinders. Arch. Environ. Health. 51(3): 175–176, 1996.

72. Sternglass, E. J. Evidence for low-level radiation effects on the human embryo and fetus. Hanford Radiobiology Symposium. Radiation Biology of the Fetal and Juvenile Mammal, Sikoff, M. R., Mahkum, D. S., Eds. U.S. Atomic Energy Commission. Symposium 17. pp. 693–716. 1969.

73. Schneider, K. Scientist who managed to 'shock the world' on atomic workers' health. New York Times. p. A-11. May 3, 1990.

74. Mangano, J. J. Cancer mortality near Oak Ridge, Tennessee, Internat. J. Health Services. 24(3): 521–533, 1994.

75. Sternglass, E. J., Gould, J. M. Breast cancer: Evidence for a relation to fission products in the diet. Internat. J. Health Serv. 23(4): 783–804, 1993.

76. Rosenthal, H. L. Accumulation of Sr-90 in teeth of children. Radiation Biology of the Fetal and Juvenile Mammal. Proceedings of the 9th Annual Hanford Biology Symposium. Sikov, R. R., Mahlum, D. D., Eds. AEC Symposium Vol. 16. pp. 163–172. 1969.

77. Jablon, S., Hrubec, A., Boice, J. D. Cancer in populations living near nuclear facilities. J. Amer. Med. Assoc. 265(11): 1403–1408, 1991.

78. Gould, J. M., Sternglass, E. J. Cancer mortality near U.S. nuclear reactors. 100 Jahre Roentgen: Medizinische Stahlenbelastung Bewertung des Risikos. Gesellschaft fur Stahlenschutz. pp. 233–250. 1995.

79. Howe, G. R. Risk of cancer mortality in populations living near nuclear facilities. J. Amer. Med. Assoc. 265(11): 1438–1439, 1991.

80. Sternglass. Op. cit., 1971.

81. Gould, J. M., Goldman, B. A. Deadly Deceit: Low-Level Radiation High-Level Cover-Up. Four Walls, Eight Windows. New York. 266 pages. 1991.

82. Ibid., p. 797.

83. Richardson, R. B., Eatough, J. P., Henshaw, D. L. Dose to red bone marrow from natural radon and thorium exposure. Brit. J. Radiol. 64: 608–624, 1991.

84. Sternglass, E. J. Personal communication. 11-11-94.

85. Sternglass and Gould. Op. cit., 1993.

86. Westin, J. B., Richter, E. The Israeli breast cancer anomaly. In: Davis, D. L., Hoel, D., Eds. Trends in Cancer Mortality in Industrial Countries. Ann. N.Y. Acad. Sci. 609: 269–279, 1990.

87. Aamodt, N. O. Analysis of cancer mortality in Pennsylvania as a result of the operation of the TMI nuclear generating plants and the nuclear accident at TMI-Unit-2. p. 10. December 7, 1987.

88. Wasserman, H. The disaster at Three Mile island is not over. Utne Reader. 34–44, Nov./Dec. 1987.

89. Wing, S., Richardson, D., Armstrong, D., Crawford-Brown, D. A reevaluation of cancer incidence near the Three Mile Island nuclear plant: The collision of

evidence and assumptions. Environ. Health Perspect. 105(1): 52–57, 1997.

90. Wasserman. Op. cit., p. 44.

91. Interim Report of the Advisory Committee on Human Radiation Experiments. Appendix B, 3(2). October 21, 1994.

> On the Committee were the following:
> Secretary Hazel O'Leary, Department of Energy
> Secretary William Perry, Department of Defense
> Attorney General Janet Reno
> Secretary Donna Shalala, Department of Health and Human Services
> Secretary Jesse Brown, Department of Veterans Affairs
> Director Alice Rivlin, Office of Management and Budget
> Director James Woolsey, Central Intelligence Agency
> Administrator Daniel Goldin, National Aeronautics and Space Administration

92. Ibid., pp. 17, 18.

93. Ibid., pp. 38, 39. The destruction of the CIA data was ordered by Richard Helms, then Director. Perhaps the most alarming is the CIA MKULTRA program, which was "concerned with research and development of chemical, biological, and radiological materials capable of employment in clandestine operations to control human behavior" (p. E-1.2) and "CIA secretly provided funding for the construction of a wing of Georgetown University Hospital in the 1950s so that it would have a locale to carry out clinical testing of its biological and chemical programs. Dr. Charles F. Geschickter, a Georgetown doctor who conducted cancer research and experimented with radiation therapy, acted as cover for CIA financing." (Ibid., p. E-1.3.)

94. Burns, R. U.S. studied radiation weapon in 1940s for civilian targets. Washington Post. p. A-13. December 27, 1994.

95. Senator John Glenn, News Release. December 1, 1994.

96. Gofman, J. W. News release. A prime cause of breast cancer: What did we know, and when did we know it? February 22, 1994.

97. Murphy, K. Emergency response failed after chemical blast at nuclear site, study concludes. Washington post. p. A-12. July 27, 1997.

98. Sternglass, Gould. Op. cit., 1993.

99. Sherman, J. D. Structure-activity relationships of chemicals causing endocrine, reproductive, neurotoxic and oncogenic effects—A public health problem. Toxicol. Indust. Health. 10(3): 163–179, 1994.

100. Edwards, M., Ludwig, G. Soviet pollution, and Chernobyl. National Geographic. 186(2): 70–99, 100–115, 1994.

7

HORMONES ONE
HUMAN AND ANIMAL
PHARMACEUTICALS

What are human beings without animals?
If all animals ceased to exist, human beings would die of a great
loneliness of the spirit. For whatever happens to the animals will happen
also to human beings. . . . All things connect."
—Said Chief Seattle

It is becoming more and more clear that ionizing radiation and biologically
active chemicals are partners in crime. Major risk factors in the development
of breast cancer are estrogenic hormones. Too much estrogen; estrogen too
soon, as during a young girl's development; inappropriate timing of estrogen
exposure; and the wrong kinds of estrogen are factors in this breast cancer
epidemic.

You may rightfully ask: "I never took hormones. Why should I be concerned
about them?" The answer is, you may not have *taken* hormones, but you may
have been *dosed* with hormones, most likely without your knowledge or your
consent, as a result of medications you were given, or in foods that you ate.

Why would anyone produce synthetic hormones? On the surface a number
of the products appear to answer a panoply of needs, and despite known negative effects on human and animal health, they have been approved by the
FDA for a number of medical "ills," and sanctioned by the Agriculture
Department as animal growth agents.

One of the most widely used of the synthetic hormones is diethylstilbestrol, also called DES. DES was prescribed to women to prevent miscarriage,
to treat post- menopausal "complications," to "cure" headaches, dizziness,

nervousness, depression, frigidity, insomnia, muscle and joint pains, vaginitis (including gonorrhea), and infertility; and it was taken to prevent conception. DES was administered to food animals to promote weight—actually, fat—gain. Subsequently, we consumed the meat of cattle, swine, and poultry that had been dosed with DES.

DES was and is easy and cheap to manufacture, affording large profits to those companies that sell it. As a consequence, before it was finally banned from much of the meat supply, DES became administered to nearly the entire United States population.

The failure to prevent the use of these chemicals, and now remedy the problems resulting from synthetic estrogenic compounds in the environment, is not because of lack of knowledge. The history of the development of synthetic estrogens such as DES with its enormous commercial value has been known for decades. Understanding these historical developments is basic to understanding the development of today's epidemic of hormonally related cancers, and may help illuminate the enormous power, pressure, and profits behind this industry.

A CENTURY OF KNOWLEDGE

In a series of three lectures, delivered in 1892, the link between cancer and exposure to soot, tars, and paraffins was first described. Those affected were mainly young chimney sweeps who developed cancer of the scrotum.[1] This was the result of skin contact with carcinogenic chemicals in the soot and tars. These young men had little access to soap, water, and clean clothes, thus the chemicals remained in intimate contact with the skin of their bodies. Later, experimenters noticed that extracts from peat, brown coal, lignite, coal tar, and petroleum possessed estrogenic activity of varying orders.

By 1934 the English doctors Cook and Dodds showed estrogenic activity in at least eight different forms of stilbenes derived from tars.[2] Figure 7.1 shows the simple stilbene "skeleton" upon which are added chemical "arms" to produce other chemicals. Adding arms does not alter greatly the basic action, but may change the potency, and not incidentally, the patentability of a compound so created.

It was found that the simplest of the stilbenes, dihydroxystilbene, gave an estrogenic response.[3] But the diethylstilbestrol form of the chemical, DES,

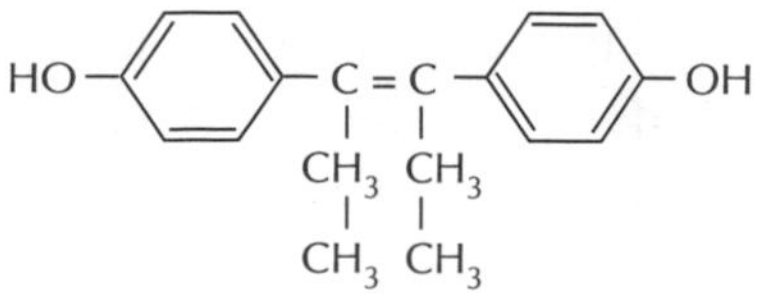

Figure 7.1
Diethylstilbestrol (DES) and stilbene molecules

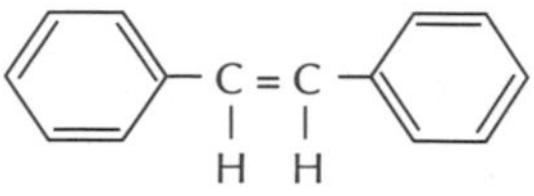

showed activity 400 times greater than that of any natural estrogen, lending itself to commercial development.[4]

My research took me to the beautiful, wood-paneled library of the British Museum. There with dusty volumes, not checked out for decades, I read that the discoverers themselves, Cook and Dodds, cautioned: "In view of the fact that many such materials are known to contain carcinogenic constituents, the clinical use of such extracts without very stringent refinement is scarcely to be entertained."[5]

Despite this august warning, synthetic hormonal products were developed and their commercial development continues today. Over half a century ago, experimenting with estrogenic chemicals, researchers produced cancer of the breast[6] and testicles[7] in laboratory animals. Rabbits dosed with DES developed proliferation of breast cells and ducts, simulating human cystic mastitis, and also developed genital cancers.[8]

Noted early was the effect of *intermittent* exposure, producing estrogenic changes in the uterus and vagina, and inducing puberty in immature animals.[9] A cycle of but two days produced the highest breast cancer incidence in male mice.[10] It is this intermittency that is important to understand in the context of cancer: nearly all human carcinogenic exposures are intermittent, turning on or turning off vital functions, until at one point in time, reversibility ceases.

COMMERCIAL DEVELOPMENT OF DES AND OTHER HORMONES

Synthetic estrogens, manufactured from coal-tar and petroleum products, were easily produced. British, European, and American chemical companies became involved in the development and promotion of estrogen products. DES, hexestrol, and dipropionate forms of the stilbene-based chemicals became commercially available by 1934.

By 1939, it was known that DES differed from the natural estrogen in three important ways: DES was not readily inactivated; deposits remained in the body; and DES was excreted intact in the feces and urine—three factors contributing to the load of hormonally active chemicals in the environment. Seldom considered, these excretion products in sewage can remain active in water, soil, and sediment, affecting other species, and be absorbed by plants and animals that have fat stores.

The American Drug Manufacturing Association convened a meeting in Washington, D.C., to "decide what procedure would quickest and most effectively satisfy the Food and Drug Administration with regard to stilbestrol." At the meeting, held on January 28, 1941, at the Hotel Washington were the following representatives and their respective companies:

Dr. D. C. Hines	Eli Lilly
Drs. J. A. Norrell and Church	Squibb
Drs. F. J. Stockman and J. B. Rice	Winthrop Chemical
Dr. J. M. Carlisle	Merck
Mr. Edgar Carter	Abbott Laboratories
Dr. W. Gifford Upjohn	Upjohn
Dr. W. A. Feirer	Sharp and Dohme
Mr. Ambrose Hunsberger, Jr.	Wyeth
Dr. E. Losinski	Charles E. Frost and Co.
Mr. Hutchinson	Ayerst, McKenna and Harrison, Ltd.

In attendance as well was Mr. Carson P. Frailey of the American Drug Manufacturers Association, the forerunner of today's Pharmaceutical Manufacturers Association, recently renamed the Pharmaceutical Research and Manufacturers of America.

There was concern among those present at the 1941 meeting that "certain clinicians in New York City seem to be the only ones opposing the release of stilbestrol at the present time and it was felt that if the evidence furnished by other clinicians could all be presented to them they might alter their stands. Drs. Stockman and Dr. Rice (Winthrop Chemical Co.) reported some success in this direction already in the case of Dr. Ephraim Shorr."[11] It was the knowledge and concern by Dr. Shorr, along with Drs. Robinson and Papanicolaou who had cautioned against the use of DES.

DES AND GENITAL CANCERS

As early as 1939, DES was found to cause changes in the cells of the genital tract.[12] That research had been supported by the Rockefeller Foundation and carried out at the Sloan Hospital for Women in New York City, forerunner of the cancer treatment hospital, Memorial Sloan-Kettering, the latter named for the head of General Motors.

During the same year, and in the same city, and again sponsored by The Rockefeller Institute for Medical Research, another group of researchers concluded that "stilbestrol (DES) in its present form is not suitable for the human being."[13] One of the three authors was the developer of the smear test to diagnose genital cancer, Dr. Papanicolaou, after whom the "Pap test" is named.*

Liver toxicity in animals and nausea in women were findings of concern impeding the commercialization of DES. Nobel prize winner Dr. Hans Selye, from Montreal, described abnormal liver changes as well as a high rate of mortality among mice treated with DES. He said: "It is well for the physician to realize that oestrogens do not only affect the sex organs but have general systemic effects, and that weight per weight, diethylstilbestrol proved more toxic in the majority of our experiments than the natural estrogens."[14]

Drug companies pressured the medical establishment to negate and deflect criticism in order to get products approved. Plans to obtain human information regarding liver toxicity and nausea were arranged to use the findings of Dr. Manuel Soule, consultant endocrinologist to the Department of Obstetrics and Gynecology at Washington University in St. Louis. Thus began a bizarre and inhumane experiment.

---

*Note: Development of a variety of cancers from a single form of a chemical is similar to the action of other carcinogens. For example, the asbestos-caused cancers were neither "site specific" nor of a single biological type. Asbestos-related cancers occurred in the chest, in the abdominal cavity, and were represented by malignancy in all three cell types. So too has DES caused cancers at many different sites: breast is but one. Others include ovary, vagina, uterus, testis, and kidney.

Eli Lilly's Dr. Hines wrote: "It was ascertained that Dr. Soule has access to a ward at the St. Louis City Hospital where relatively large numbers of incurable cancer patients are cared for. The percentage of autopsies on this service is very high and Dr. Soule will be glad to undertake the administration of large quantities of stilbestrol to some of these patients with the idea of studying the livers at autopsy. We will forward him a supply of the 25 mg. capsules which are being prepared for use in toxemia of pregnancy."[15]

Hines' strategy to negate reports of nausea associated with DES was to "demonstrate that the undesirable side-effects of stilbestrol are also produced by the natural estrogens, and if it can be shown that stilbestrol is no more toxic than they, there can be no legitimate reason for withholding the drug from the market."[16] No mention was made as to the ethics of imposing the burden of nausea upon the St. Louis Hospital patients already sick and dying of cancer. It was "clinic" patients, translated as poor, who became the ones for experimental study.

In another experiment, Winthrop Chemical Co. supplied DES for use at the Hutchinson Memorial Clinic at Tulane University in New Orleans. Often, describing the patients as "clinical material" is a strategy to render a person an object, less than human. Women as young as 20 years of age were administered DES for such symptoms as "headache, dizziness, nervousness, hot flashes, depression, muscle and joint pains, frigidity, insomnia, vaginitis and irritability."[17] What was the ultimate health experience of these unwitting women? There are no follow-up studies.

By 1943, Dr. Karl John Karnaky, of Baylor and Jefferson Davis Hospital, Houston, boasted of having given DES to more than 800 women.[18] A year later, his total was 3227 people, including 86 children ages 2 to 12. He included "a negro girl, fourteen years of age" who was given a cumulative dose of 17,783 mg of DES over a 15-month period.[19] Her ultimate fate, like the fate of all the Karnaky patients, remains unknown.

In 1941, the FDA approved the release of DES into commerce, despite documented adverse effects upon multiple body systems. Early DES studies, which produced breast cancer in animals,[20,21] was carried out under the auspices of the National Cancer Institute. These findings were evidently ignored by the Food and Drug Administration when it approved DES for use on women. Low cost and high profit may have been significant factors in the promotion of DES: 0.5 mg of stilbestrol cost less than 2 cents to make.[22]

Table 7.1

EARLY CORPORATE INVOLVEMENT IN HORMONE PRODUCTION, RESEARCH, CLINICAL TRIALS, AND PROMOTION

Pharmaceutical Co.	Country	Year
Boots Pure Drug Co, Ltd.	England	1934
Ayerst	USA	1939
British Drug Houses Ltd.	England	1939
Society of Chemical Industry in Basel (CIBA)	Switzerland	1939
George A. Breon & Co.	USA	1945
Glaxo	England	1942
Harrison	USA	1939
Lederle	USA	1945
McKenna	USA	1939
Merck	Germany/USA	1939
Ortho	USA	1942
Parke Davis	USA	1942
Schering	USA	1939
Squibb & Sons	USA	1939
Wallace & Tiernan Products	USA	1943
White Laboratories	USA	1945
Winthrop	USA	1942

While Eli Lilly Corporation had a major investment in DES, it was by no means the only corporation with interest in the drug. Worldwide, those involved in DES production and promotion included nearly every major pharmaceutical firm. See Table 7.1.

"ACCIDENTS" OF PREGNANCY AND THE DES DAUGHTERS (AND SONS)

Promoting the use of DES during pregnancy in the face of mounting evidence of toxicity, Karnaky stated: "Stilbestrol will be used as a routine in all obstetrical cases," and "we can give too little stilbestrol but we cannot give too much."[23] The DES given by Karnaky to women and their offspring was supplied by Ortho Products, Inc., E. R. Squibb and Co., and Parke Davis & Co.[24]

Despite corroborating reports against the use of DES, which cited nausea, elevation of cholesterol, and darkening of the breasts of babies born to mothers who had been give stilbestrol (an ominous sign of estrogen stimulation in the fetus), representatives at Eli Lilly submitted their application to FDA in 1947, proposing the use of stilbestrol for the prevention of toxemia of pregnancy and to prevent abortion.[25] Such use in women was proposed, despite findings that one form of stilbestrol caused abortion in cattle.[26]

Clinical experiments were cited to show the "harmlessness of the drug," despite other reports of ill effects and, most importantly, the ineffectiveness of DES to alter the course of pregnancy.[27,28] If any of the mothers developed cancer, or their children developed genital abnormalities or cancers, we shall never know. There are no follow-ups in the literature on women defined as "experimental subjects" and "clinical materials."

Despite 15 years of reports demonstrating cancer and other adverse effects in both humans and animals, Drs. Olive and George Smith, a wife and husband team from Harvard Medical School, using Squibb-supplied DES, pressed on with clinical studies, administering DES to pregnant women, in an attempt to prevent "fetal wastage."[29] One might expect that women who had previously miscarried would be the object of their research but that was not the case. The Smiths stated: "women in their first pregnancies were chosen to compose our largest homogeneous series in which the prophylactic value of stilbestrol was investigated in relation to the complications of late pregnancy."[30]

Across Boston, at the New England Deaconess and Massachusetts Memorial hospitals, Drs. Meissner, Sommers, and Sherman, concerned about the uterine disease they were finding in women who had been treated with "depot" estrogens during pregnancy, tested DES on animals. The DES-dosed rabbits developed the same genital diseases—polyps, hyperplasia, metaplasia, and cancer—that had been diagnosed in the DES-dosed women.[31]

Thirteen more years elapsed before Drs. Herbst and Scully, two Harvard physicians, reported an extremely rare form of vaginal cancer that had occurred in seven young women, only 15 to 22 years of age.[32] The next year, the link between maternal DES exposure and cancer in their daughters was definitely confirmed.[33,34]

In the decade before 1970, approximately 1 million or more pregnant women were given DES. Added to the burden of cancer and reproductive dysfunction were immune system disorders and depression.[35] On one level, unequivocal knowledge of this hormone's ability to cause harm was consistently ignored. On another level there was an abandonment of ethics: those unfortunate women who were the subject of "clinical trials" were never systematically followed up. Thus is the legacy of the DES daughters. Affected too were DES sons, who like their female counterpart, have developed genital abnormalities and cancers.

CONTRACEPTION AND LACTATION

In 1971, the same year that DES was identified as a human carcinogen, it was being touted by the directors of student health services at the University of Alberta in Canada, and at the University of Michigan in the United States, as a contraceptive.[36] DES was touted to be sufficiently effective that it could "turn a Friday night indiscretion into a Monday morning routine appointment rather than a week-end emergency."[37]

Critical of physicians who prescribed hormonally active drugs in an uncontrolled manner, the Senate Subcommittee on Health, chaired by Senator Edward Kennedy, held hearings where witnesses stated that perhaps 2 million women had been given DES for contraceptive purposes. A consultant to the American Association for the Advancement of Science's communications program for the Public Understanding of Science wrote: "doctors will continue to be able to freeboot their way around the pharmacopeia—at the expense, as one witness put it, 'of the captive human guinea pigs represented by college students, prisoners and the poor.'"[38] Despite the passage of some 25 years, this has not changed.

Given the dire consequences of DES-induced cancer, and what was known at the time, one could question the responsibility of medical journals printing articles about the contraceptive use of DES, rather than discouraging its use. Unfortunately, 2 years later, the unapproved use of DES for contraceptive purposes was still being reported.[39]

Less known is the use of DES and chemicals similar to DES to suppress lactation in women who, following delivery, did not breast feed their infants. Such research, to promote the use of DES, was supported by the manufacturers from 1939 to the early 1940s.[40,41] Despite documentation showing ineffectiveness of estrogens versus a nonactive placebo in preventing breast engorgement,[42] these products and recommendations continue in commerce today. The simple procedure of wearing a snug-fitting brassiere and using ice packs will suppress lactation, avoiding unnecessary and costly drugs. There are no follow-up reports of women given DES or other synthetic estrogens to suppress lactation. Women who were administered DES postpartum will not know if it was that event that set in motion the breast cancer that developed years later. The total number of women exposed to DES, during prenatal life to adulthood, from the time of its development in the early 1930s to date, is incalculable.

HORMONES AND THE CULT OF BIG BREASTS

In 1940, two male stilbestrol workers were diagnosed with a "dangerous" type of cellular growth of their breasts.[43] Infants and children did not escape the unwanted effects, developing breast growth as a result of skin absorption of DES.[44] The use of estrogen-containing vaginal creams,[45] and estrogen-containing hair lotions, causes enlargement of the breasts, called gynecomastia.[46] The skin is not a barrier to the passage of hormonally active chemicals, but a rather ready route of absorption for such fat-soluble chemicals as these. In an effort to promote breast enlargement, estrogens were incorporated into skin cremes and advertised in the pulp magazines of the 1940s and 1950s. We have no way of knowing how many women, believing in a quick fix for a pinup figure, later developed breast cancer.

Statistics as to the rates of breast cancer in employees of pharmaceutical manufacturing plants who handle hormonally active chemicals such as birth control pills, estrogen-replacement products, or other similar products are woefully absent.

That estrogens, however administered, orally or though the intact skin, have a profound effect upon the human breast is not in dispute. Stimulation of breast growth and breast cancer from both natural and synthetic chemicals was described early on.[47-49] What is of concern is the headlong rush for the commercial development and promotion of estrogenic and other hormonal products without considering their contribution to the burden of cancer, and the hormonal load upon the population and upon the environment. Still, today there is no plan nor concerted effort to clean up the already excessive load of hormonally active chemicals in the biosphere.

DESIGNER FARM ANIMALS

DES became a major food additive, used in dairy cattle to increase milk production, and in steers, swine, and poultry to increase weight, despite reports of adverse effects upon the animals.[50] When administered to male chicks, DES has a caponizing (castration) effect.[51] Despite the finding that DES caused stimulation of the genital tracts of female chicks,[52] it still resulted in large-scale use. DES, at a cost of a cent to a cent-and-a half for each bird, was promoted to fatten both chickens and cockerels to upgrade an entire market.[53] That DES caused the undesirable side effect of weight gain when given to women[54] did not stop the widespread use of DES in the agricultural industry. As early as *1947,* a hormonal effect was demonstrated in women who *consumed* poultry treated with DES![55] Even today, we have no idea what portion of undesirable weight gain results from hormonal agents in our food supply.

Not only was the information concerning adverse effects ignored, but Eli Lilly, a major producer of DES, "captured the stilbestrol food market."[56] The FDC reported: "Lilly's Stilbosol Premix, diethylstilbestrol cattle feed additive, is now being fed to about 68% of the 10 million cattle annually fattened up for slaughter in this country," according to officials of the company's Agricultural Products Division who were quoted in an *Agricultural Age* (*Ag Age*) "success" story telling how Lilly broke into an entirely new market. Within 90 days after the premix was first marketed in December 1954, it was being fed to 38% of the cattle being fattened for slaughter, and *Ag Age* quoted Lilly officials as hoping to eventually gain 85% of this market."[57]

Despite accumulating knowledge of adverse effects, corporate-sponsored research continued apace at a number of agricultural schools to promote the use of DES in the food supply.[58] There has never been a systematic effort to determine the extent of distribution of this chemical in feed stocks, in commerce, or in pharmaceuticals.

There was an additional aspect to DES, the bizarre facts of which were played out before the U.S. Congress, called the "Mink Hearings."[59] Because mink are meat-eaters, it became the practice to feed these fur-bearing animals on wastes from poultry slaughter houses. These wastes contained not only meat, but pellets of fat-promoting, hormonally active DES that had been inserted into the necks of the birds. Female mink, fed as little as 0.00007% DES in their food failed to produce kits, with indication of "permanent damage ... to the reproductive organs of growing mink."[60] As if this were not bad enough, the DES-fed mink developed thickened skin with absence of hair in patches. And they were fat. Now there's a picture: a bald, fat, sterile mink!

At the Congressional hearings, testimony was given as to the way in which DES had been tested on humans. Testifying before Congress, Dr. Enders from Swarthmore College said: "I am definitely opposed to the use of diethyl-stilbestrol in any form, and I would not use any poultry myself for my family that had diethylstilbestrol in it."[61]

One would have thought such statements and the effects observed in mink would have been translated into public health policy, but Dr. Byerly from the Bureau of Animal Industry of the U.S. Department of Agriculture responded to Dr. Enders' opinion by canceling a grant of $5000, which had been awarded to support Dr. Enders' research. Despite a Congressional appropriation of nearly $2 million, Byerly defended the grant cancellation on the basis of "saving money."

In regard to the DES-laced poultry, who among the general public was as informed as Dr. Enders? As of 1971, it was estimated that of 40,000,000 cattle slaughtered yearly, three-quarters of them had been treated with DES.[62] How many hundreds of thousands of us consumed those DES-laced broilers, chickens, capons, and beef cattle?

What contribution DES has played in the population developing cancer will never be known. A prudent person would believe that the Congressional "Mink Hearings" would have resulted in regulatory action by the Food and Drug Administration and by the Department of Agriculture. Unfortunately, it took *twenty-two* more years to ban DES from the food supply.

And it took another Congressional Hearing to reveal that the FDA had rejected its own Advisory Panel on Carcinogenesis and had delayed the removal of DES from the food supply.[63] More than a decade later, despite more than adequate proof of a link to cancer, tax-supported research into the use of DES in cattle was still being done.[64]

A recent book raises concerns about the possibility of an industry effort to reintroduce DES for cattle. After noting: "In the battle over DES as a carcinogen, 'science could never prove a negative, and scientists could never guarantee safety,'" the reviewer adds "no one ever found that DES administered to cattle caused a single case of cancer in humans."[65,66]

Returning to the issue of human disease, while DES was finally banned in 1979, it is recommended that a thorough history in regard to beef and poultry consumption should be obtained from every woman who has developed breast cancer. This is especially important in women who report early menarche and/or late menopause, both signs of estrogenic stimulation.

In the United States, not only breast cancer, but obesity are major public health problems. It is the practice to blame the overweight person for poor eating habits, while at the same time allowing the use of hormonal agents in the production of meat. With DES banned, other drugs are allowed to promote the growth of meat animals. These are anabolic hormones, designed to increase growth and muscle bulk, while incidentally increasing food intake. What effects these hormonal agents have on breast cancer, obesity, prostatic cancer, hypertension, heart disease, high cholesterol, and other illnesses are largely unknown to the public, and the public has not demanded answers.

As recently as 1998, Eli Lilly Co. was selling DES for treatment of breast cancer in "appropriately selected women and men with metastatic disease," and for treatment of advanced prostate cancer.[67] There are no studies reporting the results from treatment with DES versus other treatments relative to survival. Given that the purpose of using DES is its estrogenic effect, prescribing DES to a man with prostatic cancer is to negate the man's own male hormones. One might question the wisdom of giving a toxic and carcinogenic product to a man or woman already burdened with cancer.

DES, DOSE AND PERSISTENCE

DES and its chemical cousins are unlike natural estrogens. Natural estrogens are readily metabolized and excreted from the body. The synthetic estrogens remain deposited at the site of injection and are poorly metabolized, resulting in large amounts of unchanged, active chemicals being excreted in the urine and feces.[68] This latter factor is important because even sewage that has passed through a treatment facility contains active chemicals in the discharge. These can be taken up by fish; birds and animals that eat the fish; into fat-containing plants; into the animals that graze on the plants; and ultimately into the human food supply. Thus, a cycle of exposure and reexposure is set in motion.

Intermittent dosing of fat-soluble chemicals produces a *reservoir* of exposure, as when a chemical is retained in the body's fat stores and/or is slowly excreted. Such intermittency of dose and retention within the body are a critical factors in carcinogenic activity. The daily—and repeated—intake of a chemical that takes a year or more to excrete means there is a gradual accumulation of that chemical within a person's body. It follows that chemicals, slowly released and fat-soluble, become concentrated in the fat stores of the body, available to wreak their harm.

As an example, a daily intake of 1/100 milligram (0.01 mg) of chemical "X" that takes a year to be excreted from the body means that at the end of a month, 30 times 0.01 mg, or 0.30 mg, has accumulated.

Scientists speak of "half-life" of a chemical, referring to the length of time for half of the chemical or product under question to leave the body. Lipid-soluble chemicals possessing hormonal actions, such as DES, polychlorinated biphenyls (PCBs), dioxins, and the pesticide DDT are retained in the body for up to decades, long enough to do their biological damage.

The lower incidence of breast cancer in vegetarians and in certain European countries that have banned the importation of United States hormone-treated beef may be one of the keys to the United States cancer epidemic. But, while eliminating one source of contamination, persons who eat fish from contaminated waters may increase their load of hormonally active chemicals.

Lest the public believe that the food supply became hormone-free with the banning of DES, it was but one of *ten* hormones the FDA permitted in food at that time. Although the list of specific chemicals permitted in food has changed with time, hormones are never absent from the list. Conscious avoidance of pharmaceutical DES is one thing, but deliberate contamination of the food supply is another. We are not yet free from the effects of this particular agricultural/pharmaceutical practice.

Years of research has demonstrated that DES has the capacity to cause cancers at many different sites: breast, ovary, vagina, uterus, testis, and kidney. This information has been ignored to our collective peril. With the promotion of tamoxifen, a chemical cousin of DES, for the treatment of breast cancer, understanding of the action of these chemicals has never been more critical.

BOVINE GROWTH HORMONE

Neither Eli Lilly with its growth hormone Optiflex, nor Monsanto with Posilac, its bovine growth hormone, appears to have lessened their efforts to push drugs for the food supply.[69,70] Again, we do not know the long-term effects of these artificial hormones upon the population.

In 1994, the FDA granted Monsanto permission to manufacture and promote recombinant bovine growth hormone (rBGH) for dairy herds, with the dubious rationale that the cows will produce more milk. It may become one of the biggest FDA-approved experiments on human health that has been done since DES was approved. There are no longer any identifiable control groups, not exposed to rBGH, with which to make any comparisons since nearly everyone in the United States is drinking hormone-laced milk and eating rBGH-contaminated yogurt, dairy-cow-derived hamburgers, sour cream, cream cheese, butter, cheese, and other processed foods, from baked goods to baby formula. Only those who totally avoid dairy products have been spared this exposure. While some consumers have access to milk products from dairies certifying no use of rBGH, most consumers do not, especially those buying products from mixed-herd cooperatives.

This genetically engineered food product went on sale in February 1994 after final approval by the FDA—despite opposition from the American Public Health Association[71] and countless consumer's groups in the United States.[72] The fact that rBGH is banned in Norway, Sweden, Denmark, the Netherlands, and parts of Canada has not stopped its use in the United States.

To make the synthetic product, drug companies learned to remove the tiny portion of cow-DNA that codes for this hormone, combine it with the DNA from a bacteria that grows in the intestine, called *E. coli,* and grow the bacteria in vats and then extract the rBGH. Originally four chemical/drug companies developed bovine growth hormone: Monsanto, American Cynamid, Upjohn, and Eli Lilly.[73] While Monsanto controls the United States market, Lilly's hormone, Optiflex (somidobove), is marketed by its Elanco division in the Czech Republic, Mexico, and the Soviet Union.[74]

Monsanto Corporation's introduction of its product, called Posilac, prompted opposition from consumers who wanted the product banned until a number of safety questions had been resolved. Early requests to have milk labeled when it comes from rBGH-treated cows was largely unsuccessful. Monsanto opposed such labeling, and so far, only a few states, Vermont and Wisconsin among them, along with a few dairy farms, have had the courage to buck such a powerful corporation.

The U.S. FDA sided with Monsanto and opposed labeling of milk as free of rBGH. Monsanto filed two lawsuits against milk processors who labeled their product as rBGH-free, arguing a label would imply a difference that did not exist.[75] A First Amendment lawsuit, brought by anti-rBGH dairy processors against the state of Illinois and the city of Chicago was settled in favor of the processors in 1997. Products can now be labeled as rBGH-free.[76]

Despite industry claims that there is no difference between natural BGH and rBGH, they are not identical. Otherwise, cows would not develop antibodies to rBGH within the first three months of being dosed.[77] It must be assumed that the same will occur in humans. These findings raise questions about consumer health, but so far there is little information concerning human testing for reactions to rBGH, or information available to the public on rBGH in the milk supply.

A secondary issue concerning rBGH use is the development of infections in rBGH-treated cows, which leads to increased use of antibiotics and the likelihood of bacterial resistance. The Centers for Disease Control has called antibiotic resistance a "major public health crisis."[78] And, it was revealed that Monsanto itself used several unapproved drugs to control mastitis in its rBGH test herds.[79] Upjohn, with its own rBGH product, has received approval from the Department of Agriculture to use a vaccine to prevent mastitis in cattle.[80]

While there is concern for the health of dairy animals, the problems associated with infections and antibiotic usage, and a glut of milk on the market, yet another issue looms large, and that is the potential connection between rBGH and breast cancer. In a letter to Dr. David Kessler, who was Commissioner of the FDA, Samuel S. Epstein, M.D., Professor of Occupational and Environmental Medicine, expressed concern about the risk of breast cancer from consumption milk produced with rBGH. Dr. Epstein pointed out that prior to FDA approval, it was demonstrated that rBGH resulted in the release of insulin growth factor-1 (IGF-1)[81,82] that is involved in malignant transformation of normal breast epithelium. This IGF-1, released in milk, is not destroyed by pasteurization nor inactivated by digestion in the gut.

Tested in cultured human breast epithelial cells, rBGH induces uptake of IGF-1 by specific receptors in the cells, resulting in rapid cell division and multiplication, and transformation of normal human breast epithelial cells into malignant ones.[83] Dr. Epstein noted a close similarity between bovine and human IGF-1 and explained that IGF-1 is a growth factor for human breast cancer cells, functioning to maintain progression and invasiveness of malignancy. So too has IGF-1 been associated with colon cancer.

In keeping with other known adverse hormonal influences, exposure to rBGH and IGF-1 may pose the greatest risk for the young. Dr. Epstein said: "The undifferentiated prenatal and infant breast is particularly susceptible to hormonal influences. Such imprinting by IGF-I may not only constitute a direct breast cancer risk factor, but may also increase the sensitivity of the breast to subsequent unrelated risk factors," such as carcinogenic and estrogenic contaminants in food, and radiation.[84]

Six months after the introduction of Monsanto's rBGH, 8% of cows raised in the United States had received the drug.[85] Monsanto is to earn an estimated $300 to $500 million in annual income from selling rBGH, and the nation will gain an estimated 12% increase in its milk supply. But, the United

States already produces more milk than it can use, so in order to support this excess milk production, the Federal government may be required to purchase the excess milk at an additional cost to the taxpayer of $200 million. And, farmers are finding ill effects of rBGH on their herds.

It appears that the public is being enrolled in yet another massive drug experiment, without its consent and full knowledge. Without knowledge, we are denied the *right* to know which of our foods are adulterated so that we may make *informed* decisions. Given the emphasis on personal responsibility, "lifestyle," and the tendency to blame the victim, erring on the side of the drug industry seems neither fair nor wise.

Definite proof of a link between rBGH and human breast cancer is lacking at this time, but so too is definite proof of safety for women and their children. In light of the current emphasis on chemical manipulation, we consumers must become educated to protect ourselves from harm. Just now being introduced to the *consumer* are genetically altered pesticide-containing grains with little-to-no information as to their effects on humans who consume the grains and oils derived from them; on the farmers who grow them; nor the impact of pesticide resistance on other plants in the environment.[86]

Is there any wonder that hormonally related cancers are on the rise? We the people have become participants in a massing biological experiment. We were not informed, and we gave no consent. If we are to prevent more public health disasters in addition to those already known, we must become informed. If we the people perceive a threat to heath of our families and the environment, we must stop those threats by all means possible: public education, pressure on our legislators and regulatory agencies, and boycotts.

REFERENCES

1. Butlin, H. T., Cancer of the scrotum in chimney-sweeps and others. Brit. Med. J. 66–71, 1892.
2. Cook, J. W., Dodds, E. C. Proc. Royal Soc. 114B: 272, 1934.
3. Stroud, S. W. Preliminary investigation of the metabolism of stilbene. Nature. 3640: 245, 1939.
4. Dyson, G. M. A Manual of Organic Chemistry. 912–913, 918–920, Longmans, Green and Co. New York. 1940.
5. Cook, J. W., Dodds, E. C., Hewett, C. L. A synthetic oestrus-exciting compound. Nature. 56–57. 1933.
6. Lacassagne, A. Certain biological problems relating to cancer hormones and radiation. International Cancer Research Foundation. Philadelphia, PA. 1936.

7. Gordon-Taylor, T. Testicular tumors and hormones. Brit. J. Urol. 10: 1, 1938.

8. Meissner, W. A., Sommers. S. C., Sherman, G. Endometrial hyperplasia, endometrial carcinoma and endometriosis produced experimentally by estrogen. Cancer. 10(3): 500–509, 1957.

9. Cook, J. W., Dodds, E. C., Hewett, C. L, Lawson, W. The estrogenic activity of some condensed-ring compounds in relation to their biologic activities. Proc. Royal Soc. 104: 272–286, 1933/34.

10. Okey, A. B., Gass, G. H. Continuous versus cyclic estrogen administration: Mammary carcinoma in C3H mice. J. Nat. Cancer Inst. 40(2): 225-230, 1968.

11. Hines, D. C. (Eli Lilly and Co.) Trip Report. 4 pages. January 30, 1941.

12. Buxton, C. L., Engle, E. T. Effects of the use of diethylstilbestrol. J. Amer. Med. Assoc. 113(26): 2318–2320, 1939.

13. Shorr, E., Robinson, F. H., Papanicolaou, G. N. A clinical study of the synthetic estrogen stilbestrol. J. Amer. Med. Assoc. 113(2312): 2–36, 1939.

14. Selye, H. On the toxicity of oestrogens with special reference to diethylstilbestrol. Canad. Med. Assoc. J. 48–49, 1939.

15. Hines, D. C. (Eli Lilly and Co.) Report of trip to St. Louis regarding Stilbestrol. 2 pages with addendum. April 10, 1941.

16. Ibid.

17. Collins, C. G., Weed, J. C., Weinstein, B. B., Lock, F. R. Clinical experiences with stilbestrol (diethylstilbestrol). Amer. J. Obstet. Gynecol. 39(1): 117–121, 1940.

18. Abarbanel, A. R., Aranow, H., Goodfriend, M. J. Adjunctive therapy with diethylstilbestrol in obstetrics and gynecology. J. Amer. Med. Assoc. 121(14): 1123–1130, 1943. (See Abstract of the Discussion held on the paper, page 1130.)

19. Karnaky, K. J. Prolonged administration of diethylstilbestrol. J. Clin. Endocrinol. 5: 279–284, 1945.

20. Geschickter, C. F. Estrogenic mammary cancer in the rat. Readiol. 33(4): 439–449, 1938.

21. Shimkin, M. B., Grady, H. G. Carcinogenic potential of stilbestrol and estrone in strain C3H mice. J. Nat. Cancer Inst. 1: 119–128, 1941.

22. Stoddard, F. J., Metzger, I. A clinical comparison of three commercial estrogenic preparations. J. Clin. Endocrinol. 2: 209–212, 1942.

23. Karnaky, K. J. The use of stilbestrol for the treatment of threatened and habitual abortion and premature labor: a preliminary report. Southern Med. J., 35(9): 838–847, 1942.

24. Karnaky, ibid.

25. Eli Lilly and Co. New Drug Application: Diethylstilbestrol. Form FD-356, to the Food and Drug Administration, Federal Security Agency, Washington, D.C. 1 page, with 5 page attachment. April 23, 1947.

26. Folley, S. J., Watson, H. M. S. Induction of abortion in the cow by injection with stilbestrol dipropionate. Lancet. 2: 788, 1939.

27. Dieckmann, W. J., Davis, M. E., Rynkiewicz, L. M., Pottinger, R. E. Does the administration of diethylstilbestrol during pregnancy have therapeutic value? Amer. J. Obstet. Gynecol. 66(5): 1062–1081, 1953.

28. Ferguson, J. H. Effect of stilbestrol on pregnancy compared to the effect of placebo. Amer. J. Obstet. Gynecol. 65(3): 592–601, 1953.

29. Smith, G. V., Smith, O. W. Prophylactic hormone therapy. Obstet. Gynecol. 4(2): 129–141, 1954.

30. Smith, O. W., Smith, G. V. The influence of diethylstilbestrol on the progress and outcome of pregnancy as based on a comparison of treated and untreated primigravidas. Amer. J. Obstet. Gynecol. 58: 994, 1949.

31. Meissner, W. A., Sommers, S. C., Sherman, G. Endometrial hyperplasia, endometrial carcinoma, and endometriosis produced experimentally by estrogen. Cancer. 10(3): 500–509, 1957.

32. Herbst, A. L., Scully, R. E. Adenocarcinoma of the vagina in adolescence. Cancer. 25(4): 745–757, 1970.

33. Herbst, A. L., Ulfelder, H., Poskanzer, D. C. Adenocarcinoma of the vagina: association of maternal stilbestrol therapy with tumor appearance in young women. New Engl. J. Med. 285(7): 390–392, 1971.

34. Greenwald, P., Barlow, J. J., Nasca, P. C. Burnett, W. S. Vaginal cancer after maternal treatment with synthetetic estrogens. New Engl. J. Med. 285: 390–392, 1971.

35. Colborn, T., vom Saal, F. S., Soto, A. M. Developmental effects of endocrine-disrupting chemicals in wildlife and humans. Environ. Health Perspect. 101(5): 378–384, 1993.

36. Kuchera, L. K. Postcoital contraception with diethylstilbestrol. J. Amer. Med. Assoc. 218(4): 562–563, 1971.

37. Rall, M. J. The Morning-after pill. Canad. Med. Assoc. J. 125: 168, 1971.

38. Chedd, G. Illicit contraception. New Scientist. March 1, 1973.

39. Blye, R. P. The use of estrogens as postcoital contraceptive agents. Amer. J. Obstet. Gynecol. 116: 1044–1050, 1973.

40. Barnes, J. Inhibition of lactation by synthetic oestrogenic substances. Brit. Med. J. 601–603, 1942.

41. Werner, H., Joel, K. Cessation of postpartum lactation with stilbestrol. Lancet. ii: 688, 1939.

42. MacDonald, D., O'Driscoll, K. Suppression of lactation: A double-blind trial. Lancet. 623, September 25, 1965.

43. Scarff, R. W., Smith, C. P. Proliferative and other lesions of the male breast: with notes on two cases of proliferative mastitis in stilbestrol workers. Brit. J. Surg. 393–396, 1940.

44. Whittle, C. H., Lyell, A. Precocity in a girl aged 5: Due to stilbestrol inunction. Proc. Royal Soc. Med. 41(11): 760, 1948.

45. DiRaimondo, C. V., Roach, A. C., Meador, C. K. Gynecomastia from exposure to vaginal estrogen cream. New Engl. J. Med. 302: 1089–1090, 1980.

46. Gottswinter, J. M., Korth-Schutz, S., Ziegler, R. Gynecomastia caused by estrogen containing hormone hair lotion. J. Endocrinol. Invest. 7: 383–386, 1984.

47. Geschickter, C. F. Mammary carcinoma in the rat with metastasis induced by estrogen. Science. 89: 35, 1939.

48. MacBryde, C. M. The production of breast growth in the human female. J. Amer. Med. Assoc. 112: 1045, 1939.

49. Auchincloss, H., Haagensen, C. D. Cancer of the breast possibly induced by estrogenic substance. J. Amer. Med. Assoc. 114(16): 1517–1523, 1940.

50. Andrews, F. N., Beeson, W. M., Johnson, F. D. The effects of stilbestrol, dienestrol, testosterone and progesterone on the growth and fattening of beef steers. J. Animal Sci. 13(1): 99–106, 1954.

51. Jaap, R. G., Thayer, R. H. Oral administration of estrogens in poultry. Poultry Sci. 23(3): 249–251, 1944.

52. Herrick, E. H. Some influences of stilbestrol, estrone, and testosterone propionate on the genital tract of young female fowls. Poultry Sci. 23(1): 65–66, 1944.

53. Thayer, R. H., Jaap, R. G., Penquite, R. Fattening chickens by feeding estrogens. Poultry Sci. 23(6): 555, 1944.

54. Bishop, P. M. F., Boycott, M., Zuckerman, S. The oestrogenic properties of "stilboestrol" (diethyl-stilboestrol). Lancet. 1: 5–11, 1939.

55. Bird, S., Pugsley, L. I., Klotz, M. O. The quantitative recovery of synthetic estrogens from tissues of birds (gallus domesticus), the response of the birds testis, comb and epidermis to estrogen and of humans to ingestion of tissues from treated birds. Endocrinology. 40: 282–294, 1947.

56. FDC Reports. February 20, 1956.

57. FDC Reports. October 7, 1956.

58. Eli Lilly's DES feed supplement was developed at Iowa State, and Pfizer's DES ear implant was developed at Purdue University.

59. Hearings before Subcommittee No. 2, of the Committee of the Judiciary, House of Representatives, 82nd Congress. Re: H. R. 846, 1568, 2591, 2592, 2776, 2777 for the Relief of Various Mink Ranchers. March 2, 5, and 9, 1951.

60. Roberts, W. L. What happens when pellet-inserted chicken heads are fed. Amer. Fur Breeder. 23(4): 17–52, 1950.

61. Mink Hearings. p. 132.

62. Folkman, J. Transplacental carcinogenesis by stilbestrol. New Engl. J. Med. 285(7): 404–405, 1971.

63. U.S. Congressional Committee on Governmental Operations. Regulation of diethylstilbestrol (DES) and other drugs used in food producing animals. U.S. Government Printing Office. Washington, D.C. pp. 1–87, 1973.

64. Rumsey, T. S., Kozak, A. S. Tyrrell, H. F. Mineral deposition in diethylstilbestrol- and Synovex-treated steers. Beltsville Agricultural Research Center, Ruminant Nutrition Laboratory, Beltsville, MD. 49(3): 354–366, 1985.

65. Marcus, A. I. Cancer from beef: DES, Federal Food Regulation and Consumer Confidence. Johns Hopkins University Press. Baltimore. p. 235. 1994.

66. Browne, W. P. Book Reviews—The DES case. Science. 267: 394, 1995.

67. Physician's Desk Reference, Medical Economics Co. Inc. Montvale, NJ. p. 1292. 1993.

68. Zondek, B., Sulman, F. Inactivation of diethylstilbestrol by the organism. Nature. 144(3648): 596–597, 1939.

69. Eli Lilly Annual Report. 1990. In addition to Optiflex, are Rumensin, a growth-promoter for beef, Tylan, "a versatile product used to control diseases and promote growth of cattle, swine, and poultry."

70. Anon. Eli Lilly & Co. buys Monsanto drug unit, expanding to Belgium. Wall Street Journal. p. B-3. August 31, 1993.

71. Anon. The Nation's Health. APHA, Washington, D.C. p. 21. September, 1994.

72. Hansen, M., Halloran, J. M. Letter to Jerry Mande, Officer of the Commissioner, FDA, Consumer Policy Institute, Consumers Union. 7 pages. May 24, 1993.

73. Gugliotta, G. A wonder drug or threat: bovine growth hormone raises concern on milk surpluses, safety. Washington Post. p. A-3. June 24, 1990.

74. Eli Lilly Annual Report. 1990. By 1993, the product was no longer listed.

75. Anon. Monsanto sues an Iowa dairy cooperative. Washington Post. p. C-1. February 19, 1994. Montague, P., Ed. Rachel's Hazardous Waste News. #382. March 24, 1994.

76. Mothers and Others, Green Guide. 44:1, 1997. Address: 40 West 20th Street, New York, NY 10011-4211.

77. Zwickl, C. M., Smith, H. W., Tamura, R. N., Bick, P. H. Somatotropin antibody formation in cows treated with a recombinant bovine somatotropin over two lactations. J. Dairy Sci. 73(10): 2888–2895, 1990.

78. Hiss, T. "How Now, Drugged Cow?" Harper's Magazine. p. 82. October, 1994.

79. Epstein, S., Hardin, P. Confidential Monsanto Research Files Dispute Many BGH safety Claims. The Milkweed. Madison WI. 128: 306, 1990. This discusses P. J. Eppard and others, "Toxicity of CP115099 in a Prolonged Release System in Lactating Cows," Report MSL 6345. Monsanto Agricultural Co. St. Louis, MO. 1987.

80. Anon. Detroit Free Press. p. 2-E. August 27, 1993.

81. Furlanetto, R. W., DiCarlo, J. N. Somatomedin-C receptors and growth effects in human breast cells maintained in long-term tissue culture. Cancer Res. 44: 2122–2935, 1984.

82. The Merck Index. 11th Edition. Merck and Co., Inc. Rahway, NJ. p. 1373. 1989.

83. Harris, J. R., et al. Breast cancer. New Engl. J. Med. 7: 473–480, 1992.

84. Epstein, S. S. Letter to David Kessler, Commissioner, FDA. February 14, 1994.

85. Day, K. Eight percent of cows in United States given new hormone. Washington Post. p. A-12. September, 15, 1994.

86. Lappe, M., Bailey, B. Against the Grain: Biotechnology and the Corporate Takeover of Your Food. Common Courage Press. Monroe, ME. 163 pages. 1998.

8

HORMONES TOO
FALSE HORMONES

New opinions are always suspected, and usually opposed,
without any other reasons but because they are not already common.
—John Locke, English philosopher (1632–1704)

The title of this chapter, HORMONES TOO, is not a typographical error.
I use the spelling to emphasize that many products, not labeled as hormones,
not even thought of as hormones, have hormonal/endocrinal as well as
carcinogenic effects. These products and their contaminants have achieved
common usage, with little attention to their ultimate effects.

The years that brought the bulk of chemicals now threatening life on our
planet came at a time of great turmoil: economic and social unrest in Europe
that led to World War II. Undoubtedly many of the chemical "magic bullets"
helped defeat Japan and Nazi Germany, but in reality there is never just one
side to an innovation. We continue to reap those effects, both good and bad.
Understanding the history of some of these chemicals will help us to guard
against new "magic bullets" of the future.

DDT AND ITS COUSINS

It was DDT, otherwise known as dichlorodiphenyltrichloroethane, whose
insecticidal property was discovered in 1939. It was used by the military in the
early 1940s largely to eradicate malaria. Its ultimate harm and its effectiveness
in controlling insect-borne disease among the military is well documented in
Dr. John Wargo's book *Our Children's Toxic Legacy*.[1]

DDT was patented in 1944 by Geigy Corporation, the parent of CIBA-
Geigy, and promoted to agricultural interests and to the general public as a

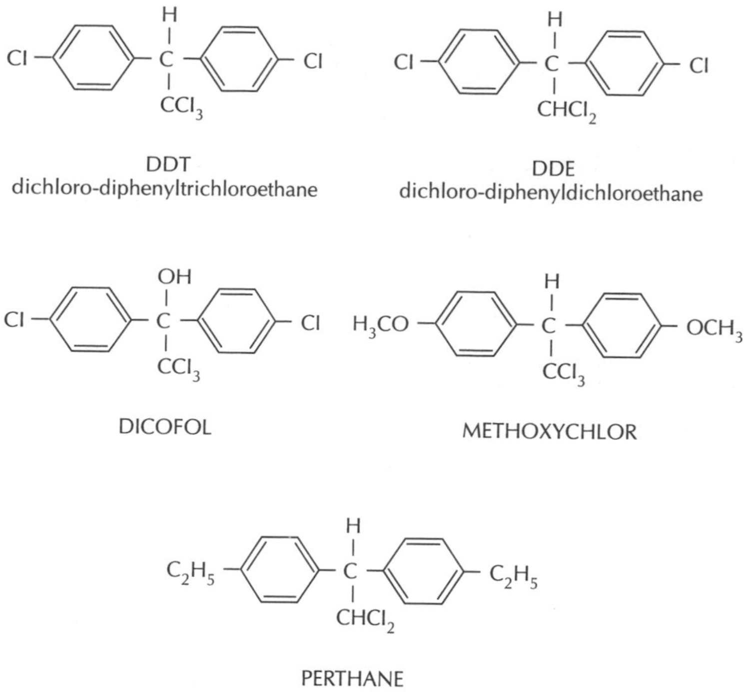

DDT
dichloro-diphenyltrichloroethane

DDE
dichloro-diphenyldichloroethane

DICOFOL

METHOXYCHLOR

PERTHANE

Figure 8.1
DDT, DDE, dicofol, methoxychlor, and perthane.

way to control insects. DDT was an effective killer: it destroyed "good" insects along with the "bad," the bees and butterflies along with the aphids, the birds and fishes along with the roaches. The arrogance of those who decide which (and who) among us living creatures are pests bears reflection, for now we humans too are succumbing to DDT's untoward effects.

Figure 8.1 shows the structure of DDT, its metabolic product DDE, and other pesticides of this organochlorine family. When one reviews the structure of DES, discussed earlier, the relationship of this "family" of pesticides to the drug DES is striking.

DDT was effective in combatting malarial mosquitoes, but the initial success was short-lived as resistant strains emerged, becoming resistant to DDT. With the passage of time and increased use of DDT, pest strains emerged, resistant not only to DDT but to many of the newly developed chemical pestic. The pesticide resistance of insects is no different from the resistance that bacteria develop when exposed to antibiotics. As the more susceptible members of a population are killed off, more resistant members remain. Eventually, their descendants cease to be affected by the pesticide or the antibiotic. Bacterial resistance has developed with devastating effects in those with tubercular and staphylococcal infections, malaria, AIDS, and many other diseases. Pesticide resistance has allowed some hardy insects to selectively increase in numbers because of an advantage over those who do not succumb to various chemicals. Widespread famine and economic upheaval are not far off if our increasingly monocultural crop practices become invaded by an insect, weed, or fungus resistant to the current chemical pesticides.

Still, during the period extending from World War II until the 1960s, DDT use expanded to nearly all foodstuffs, vegetable and animal, as well as into public, commercial, and home pest control. By 1969 a blue-ribbon U.S. Commission[2] recommended discontinuation of DDT because of its toxic effects, persistence, and insect resistance. The United States banned the use of DDT in 1972, but production of DDT and similar members of this oganochlorine family of chemicals continues worldwide. These other members of the DDT family (Figure 8.1) include the structurally related dicofol, marketed by Rhom and Haas under the name Kelthane, and methoxychlor, manufactured by Drexel Chemical Company, still used to control insects.[3]

While the organochlorine pesticides kill by poisoning the nervous system, the long-term effects of trace, sublethal exposures are more insidious, resulting in cancer and hormonal effects that interfere with both female and male reproduction.[4] Like other chemicals of this group, the organochlorine chemicals are fat-soluble, becoming stored in fat portions of the body, breast tissue included.

Human body tissues bear testimony to continuing DDT exposure. Our bodies contain measurable levels of DDT, and its two metabolic breakdown products, DDD and DDE, stored in our fatty tissues, our blood, as well as in the tissues of most of the world's fish, animals, and birds.

In 1976, the Israeli team of Marcus and Dora Wassermann and their associates found higher levels of organochlorine pesticides in the tissue of women with breast cancer.[5] United States researchers, working at three different hospitals, confirmed breast cancer associated with increased tissue levels of these pesticides, also finding PCB contamination in the same women.[6] Not only were tissue levels of pesticides increased in women with breast cancer, but blood levels of these contaminants were increased as well.[7] Still another study that compared 150 women with and without breast cancer reported no association between breast cancer and DDE/PCB levels. When the racial and ethnic groups were evaluated separately, white and African American women with breast cancer had higher levels of DDE than Asian women.[8]

It is against this background, that yet another breast cancer/organochlorine study was released. The findings of 240 women who had given blood samples between 1989 or 1990 and became diagnosed with breast cancer before mid 1992 were compared with a near-equal number of women who had not been diagnosed with breast cancer. The researchers found no difference in levels of DDE and PCBs in the women.[9]

One might have assumed that it was another equivocal or negative study being reported, but the publisher of the journal put a unique spin on the study's release, resulting in considerable media fanfare. Accompanying the report was an editorial by Stephen Safe, a researcher whose work is often funded by the Chemical Manufacturers Association,[10] who assailed "chemophobia, the unreasonable fear of chemicals, [is] a common public reaction to scientific or media reports suggesting that exposure to various environmental contaminants may pose a threat to health."[11]

Taking into consideration all the studies that measured foreign chemicals in women with breast cancer, four out of eleven studies showed a negative or equivocal connection between organochlorines in the tissues of women with breast cancer, and seven showing a positive association. Despite this, Safe added "the work of Hunter along with those of other recent studies should reassure the public that weakly estrogenic organochlorine compounds such as PCBs, DDT, and DDE are not a cause of breast cancer."[12]

More detailed analysis of the Hunter study is impeded by absence of actual data of chemical measurements; insufficient time delay to answer the question of whether 2 to 3 years after providing blood samples is a sufficient passage of time to say that women are free of breast cancer; lack of information on exposure to other estrogenic products, such as birth control pills, post-menopausal estrogenic products, other pesticides, etc.; place and condition of residence; no assessment of all the PCB congeners, but only the higher molecular weight ones;[13] no assessment of DDT; and finally, lack of discussion that DDE, the metabolic breakdown product of DDT, is not estrogenic, but anti-androgenic.[14]

The scientific article was covered by the press, and the public can thank the public relations industry for such statements as printed in the *New York Times*: "One more environmental scare bit the dust last week as scientists from the Harvard School of Public Health reported that their large and meticulous study found no evidence that exposure to the chemicals DDT and PCB's [sic] are linked to breast cancer."[15]

It is unfortunate when the press joins forces with those who fail to include the extensive scientific record, in existence for some 30 years, that demonstrates links between these chemicals and cancer, and thereby misleads an unaware public.[16] The scientific record is more extensive and compelling than what is suggested by the Hunter, Safe, and Kolata arguments.

Repeated doses of DDT, like DES, at a moderate level can result in greater total storage in the fat than a single larger dose.[17] DDT, DES, and associated organochlorines are excreted in the breast milk of all animals tested, including cows and humans.[18] This load of hormonally active chemicals are transferred via the placenta to the developing fetus, and via the milk to the nursing infant. Critical times of breast tissue development occur before birth and at the onset of menstruation. In an extensive breast cancer study, it was found that first-born women were of greater risk of breast cancer than those later in the birth order.[19] This may reflect the chemical load these first-born received during their intrauterine growth. It is unknown if there is a difference in breast cancer incidence in women who were bottle-fed as infants, as contrasted to those who were breast-fed. Transfer of chemicals to the infant follows physiologic function. Pregnancy and lactation are each pathways of excretion for the mother, with the transfer of chemicals to the developing fetus occurring at a critical time when mammary tissue is most responsive to hormonal stimulation.[20]

Official U.S. governmental surveys in the late 1970s demonstrated racial stratification of organochlorine contaminants. Adipose (fatty) tissue levels of DDT and DDE were almost twice as great in black citizens as compared to whites. Giving no comfort to any citizen, 100% of all 1000-plus human samples, black and white alike, had detectable levels of DDT and DDE.[21] PCBs also showed racial stratification, higher in blacks than whites, with fewer blacks having no contamination.[22]

But race is not the only factor. Levels of the same pesticide(s) were significantly higher in less affluent members of each race.[23] Does this reflect avoidance of toxic chemicals by persons better informed, greater use of pesticides by poorer people, or "public health" programs involving widespread pesticide use, carried out on poorer populations?

The Mantrose Company of Indonesia (close in spelling to the California

DDT manufacturer, Montrose) sells its entire production of DDT to the World Health Organization, mostly for "public health" uses in Africa.[24] Its United States forerunner, the Montrose Chemical Co., between 1949 and 1970, released into the Los Angeles sewer system an estimated 4,400,000 pounds of DDT. That's not produced or sold, but released into the environment! Sediments near the White's Point, California, sewage out-fall contain as much as 100 metric tons of technical DDT,[25] providing a ready supply for sea-dwelling creatures, and to any human who eats them.

As if the carcinogenic and hormonal effects of DDT exposure were not serious enough, 20 years ago, a U.S. governmental study demonstrated a link between these chemicals and increase in fats in the blood.[26] To my knowledge, no large-scale study has been done to determine what factor, if any, DDT or DES plays in the development of arteriosclerotic heart disease and stroke. The incidence and costs of these two illnesses are significant. Centering blame on the victim for poor eating habits has obscured this link that receives little scientific support or even consideration. Perhaps these illness are not entirely "lifestyle" after all.

DIOXINS AND DIBENZOFURANS

The Environmental Protection Agency (EPA) draft reassessment of dioxin and related compounds, released in September 1994, reaffirms not only carcinogenic properties but hormonal ones as well. Dioxins are capable of disrupting reproductive, endocrine, and immune function across multiple species.[27]

Dioxin is not a single chemical, but a family of chemicals, related by structure and action, and includes furans and polychlorinated biphenyls (PCBs). Most dioxins are formed inadvertently during manufacture of chlorinated products or during the burning of these products.

Commonly, only one of the dioxin chemicals is singled out for mention or testing. This one, tetrachlorodibenzo-*p*-dioxin, called TCDD for short, is the most toxic of the group, but by no means the only harmful member of the family. When the number of possible combinations of dioxins and furans are added together, there are 210 different forms. A short lesson in chemistry will show why. See Figure 8.2 and Table 8.1.

Why is this chemistry lesson so important? Because if only one form of dioxin is measured or considered, usually TCDD, the total biological load and

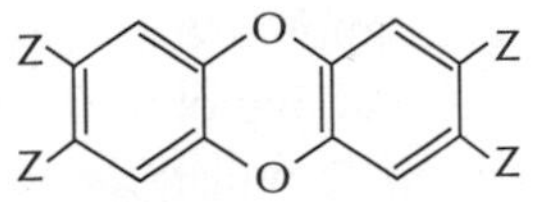

DIOXINS (In general)
Z = chlorine, bromine, or iodine

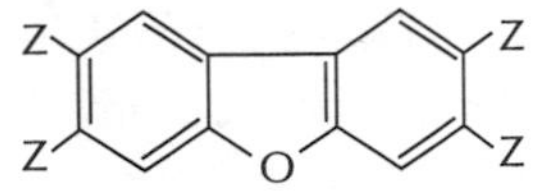

FURANS (In general)
Z = chlorine, bromine, or iodine

Figure 8.2
Chemical structure of dioxins and furans.

Table 8.1

Number of chlorine atoms	Polychlorinated dibenzodioxins — Number of isomers dioxins	Polychlorinated dibenzofurans — Number of isomers furans
Mono-	2	4
Di-	10	16
Tri-	14	28
Tetra-	22	38
Penta-	14	28
Hexa-	10	16
Hepta-	2	4
Octa-	1	1
Total	75	135

effects are greatly underestimated. And, except under controlled laboratory conditions, formation of a single dioxin or furan is not the case. Depending upon the original chemical mix, heat, presence of oxygen, etc., the production of dioxins and furans is a chance process: a witch's brew of 210 potential hazards.

The EPA has ranked the main sources of dioxins as coming from medical and municipal waste incinerators. The incinerator watchdog publication

Waste Not characterizes EPA's approach to dioxins as "Jekyll and Hyde," promoting and permitting the building of incinerators for the past 20 years, and now admitting what environmentalists and scientists have said all along, that dioxins are dangerous.

The stacks of incinerators emit not only dioxins and their cousins, the furans, but also heavy metals such as mercury, lead, cadmium, chromium, etc. Emitted also are radioactive isotopes, derived from the burning of trees and plants that have become contaminated from weapons testing and nuclear power plant fallout.[28]

EPA speaks of "acceptable risk" from these exposures. In the face of serious and irreversible effects from dioxin and radioisotope exposure, one must ask: In a democratic society, to whom are these risks acceptable and who decides? A reasonable answer is a resounding: No risk is acceptable if it is avoidable![29]

Manufactured products contaminated with dioxins and furans include Agent Orange, manufactured from the chlorinated phenoxy herbicides called 2,4-D and 2,4,5-T. The full names are 2,4-dichlorophenoxyacetic acid and 2,4,5-trichlorophenoxyacetic acid. Not only were these herbicides used in Vietnam, they were used worldwide on range lands, forests, crops, and rice fields to defoliate unwanted plant growth. 2,4-D continues for sale under many trade names and is widely used in the United States and elsewhere as "lawn care" products.

A significant site of potential dioxin contamination is in Jacksonville, Arkansas. This was the site of Vertac Chemical, run jointly by Hercules, Inc., and Uniroyal Chemical Ltd. to manufacture the herbicide Agent Orange for the Vietnam war. The U.S. EPA incinerated more than 28,000 drums of dioxins and other toxins that had accumulated at the site. In 1998, the U.S. District Court for Eastern Arkansas held the companies liable for $102 million in cleanup costs;[30] however, the companies plan to appeal, claiming it is unconstitutional to penalize a company for actions prior to the passage of the CERCLA (the Comprehensive Environmental Response, Compensation and Liability Act).[31] In other words, their argument is "if you don't make it a law to take care, then I'm not responsible." Could a private citizen, without a horde of lawyers get away with this kind of argument?

Dioxins were found as well in chlorinated phenols, many employed as antibacterial, antifungal, and preservative agents, this last including the popular wood preservative marketed as "Penta" (pentachlorophenol).

Trichlorophenol was marketed directly as Dowcide 2S for use as a fungicide and preservative. It is also a feedstock chemical used in the production of a number of pesticides and other commercial and home-use products.

Dioxins are a factor in breast cancer and in other cancers, because in part, some forms of dioxin act as hormones. Studies of several dioxins show mixed hormonal function, both estrogenic and antiestrogenic. This property is not unique to dioxins; other chemicals, notably tamoxifen, display carcinogenic, estrogenic, and antiestrogenic effects as well.

The Rotunda of the State Capitol in Harrisburg, Pennsylvania, held a display of photographs of women from each county who had developed breast cancer. I was struck by the number of nurses among the Pennsylvania Breast Cancer Coalition's group. I wondered, what combination of exposures resulted in breast cancer in these women? Was it dioxin-contaminated cleaning products, hormonally active drugs, x-ray emissions, radioisotopes in the urine, feces, and bodies of patients under their care, chemotherapy drugs, or a combination of these factors?

Unrecognized sources of hormonally active chemicals are a concern. Many women with breast cancer have never worked in heavy industry. Many women with cancer work in "clean industries," as did these nurses. Other breast cancer patients have as their primary interest homemaker, a career shared by nearly every other women, whether she works outside of her home or not. Wanting to maintain a clean and safe home, unwittingly, women have been targeted by advertisers of products containing hormonally active and carcinogenic chemicals.

HEXACHLOROPHENE

The name hexachlorophenc, marketed in the United States as pHisohex, may sound familiar.[33] Concerned about "protecting our families," and reacting to advertising hype about bacteria-killing products, many bought the concept and the products. Hexachlorophene was touted as an antibacterial agent and incorporated into soaps for both home use and on hospitalized patients. It wreaked its harm, causing brain, nerve, and liver damage.

Hexachlorophene products were used by millions of nurses and other hospital employees in the course of their work, each under the false hope of providing protection to themselves and to patients under their care. Following the death of some infants exposed to a talcum powder-hexachlorophene formulation, levels of TCDD, ranging from 20 ppt to 0.5 ppb were measured in the product.[34] Nothing is known of the nurses who handled those products.

Production workers at the Givaudan Corporation plant in Clifton, New Jersey, and at the Syntex plant in Verona, Missouri, operated by the Hoffman-Taff and North Eastern Pharmaceutical and Chemical Company, where hexachlorophene, trichlorophenols, and associated products were produced were placed in a National Institutes for Occupational Safety and Health (NIOSH) registry to study the long-term effects from dioxin exposure. Samples of trichlorophenol and hexachlorophene from the latter plant were contaminated with 67 ppb and as much as 20 ppb TCDD, the most toxic form of the dioxins; however, no information is available for total dioxin contamination.

As of 1984, approximately 6000 workers at 12 production facilities with dioxin contamination had been entered into the NIOSH registry. Unfortunately, women have been excluded from some analyses, but studies of male workers from the above two plants show "mortality from all cancers combined was 15 percent higher than expected in the overall cohort."[35] Findings in the male workers confirmed what had been known in the animal literature, where adverse hormonal effects were expressed in the hypothalamus of the brain, the pituitary, and the testicles.[36] No registry has been established for the townspeople where dioxin-contaminated plants were located, and few attempts have been made to determine the dioxin contamination in the soil, water, and food surrounding these manufacturing facilities.

We citizens have remained ignorant to the action of chemicals, acting as hormones, unintended, secretively, and with malignant results. These chemicals function like hormones, while not being directly promoted as hormones or administered as hormones. That does not mean that we have not been administered them, because indeed we have, and once in our bodies, they remain for years. The half-life of but one form of dioxin is more than 7 years.

Included in hormone-disrupting chemicals are such products as the pesticides DDT, chlordane, hexachlorobenzene, methoxychlor, and amitrole; the industrial chemicals styrene, nonylphenol, PCBs and PBBs; and the dioxins and furans, formed during the manufacture of certain chemicals, and when chlorine-containing plastics and other materials are incinerated.

Other chemicals having both estrogenic and carcinogenic actions include those called polycyclic aromatic compounds (PACs), close in structure to the natural estrogens, found naturally in tars, and produced when carbon-containing materials are burned.

As if the knowledge that many of the dioxins and furans are carcinogenic is not enough, several forms of a furan containing three chlorine atoms are "being investigated as a compound that may be clinically useful for the treatment of mammary cancer."[37] Will this be just another product, patentable and profitable, sparing the necessity of addressing remediation and primary prevention?

THE CHLORINATED PHENOLS

Living in a time of instant sound bites, and with little, or but superficial, science education for the public, we lose sight that the toxicity of many chemicals has been known for decades, and in some cases, before the turn of the century. When we fail to use past findings, we lose our ability to predict; and predictable were the adverse effects of chlorinated phenols. Four chlorinated ring-structured examples are shown in Figure 8.3.

Trichlorophenol is a common feedstock used in a myriad of chemical production processes. It was the manufacturing facility in Serveso, Italy, that blew up, where trichlorophenol was in use, contaminating the countryside

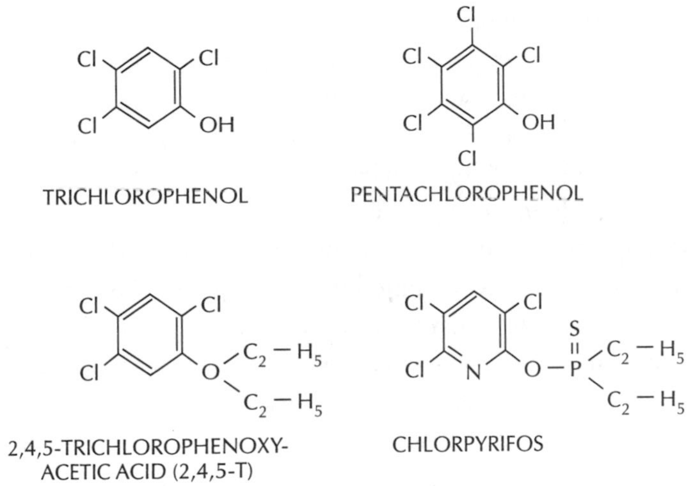

TRICHLOROPHENOL

PENTACHLOROPHENOL

2,4,5-TRICHLOROPHENOXY-
ACETIC ACID (2,4,5-T)

CHLORPYRIFOS

Figure 8.3
Chemical structure of chlorinated phenols.

with dioxins and other by-products of the production process. It is trichlorophenol that is a feedstock for the production of 2,4,5-T, half of the herbicide Agent Orange, used over Vietnam, and also used in agriculture. It is the pyridyl form of trichlorophenol that is a feedstock for the production of chlorpyrifos (Dursban), one of the most commonly used pesticides, employed in homes, schools, businesses, industry, and agriculture.[38]

The EPA has requested information from Dow Chemical Co., the producer of Dursban (chlorpyrifos), concerning possible contamination with dioxins. Information on such contamination of this widely used pesticide is in the public interest. Response to my Freedom of Information requests to the EPA produced a document that tested for a single dioxin-type chemical, and was unable to detect levels below 1 part per million.[39,40] As of this writing, it appears that this minimal information has been acceptable to the EPA.

Pentachlorophenol, better known as "Penta," is a commonly used product to treat lumber to protect against rot. Penta and its dioxin contaminants may be found on your wooden deck, the posts in your home, and on your cotton garments. The latter has occurred when "Penta" was used as a defoliant before harvesting cotton, and to prevent mildew during processing.[41]

This raises another concern when one does not consider the ramifications of technology. An ostensibly natural product, cotton, has been deemed more ecologically sound than synthetic fibers. Yet it is not the cotton that is toxic, but the process by which some cotton is harvested and processed. In attempting to cut labor costs by using chemical defoliants to remove the leaves, some cotton becomes contaminated with dioxins. The risk of dioxin contamination of this resource may not be wise. Cotton has many important uses: clothing and bedding, tampons, and baby diapers. While an industry may save money, the public will bear the risks and increased costs of human disease and ecological degradation.

Increased breast cancer was found in Finnish women exposed to the pesticide hexachlorocyclohexane (HCH)[42] and in Minnesota women who drank water contaminated with creosote.[43] Creosote, one of the end-products of oil refining, is rich in steroid-like structures called polycyclic aromatic hydrocarbons (PAHs), long known to cause breast cancer.[44]

When Percivall Pott published his findings in 1775, describing cancer of the scrotum in chimney sweeps, he was unaware that PACs were the cause. The importance of this fact is not in the link, but the 220 years it has taken for prevention to begin to be discussed openly.

THE CHLORINATED BIPHENYLS
(PCBs and PBBs)

Included in the dioxin-like chemicals are members of the biphenyl family, the polychlorinated biphenyls (PCBs), and the brominated form, called polybrominated biphenyls (PBBs). See Figure 8.4.

PCBs and PBBs, like their chemical cousins and contaminants the dioxins, may contain one or more chlorine atoms on various positions of the two basic rings. The more chlorine atoms, the longer the chemicals persist, and the more resistant they are to breakdown. But as they breakdown and release chlorine atoms, the greater is the estrogenic action.

POLYBROMINATED BIPHENYLS

Polybrominated biphenyls (PBBs) became newsworthy in the mid 1970s when between 500 to 1000 pounds of a chemical fire retardant was inadvertently combined with animal feed, resulting in the contamination of cattle, poultry, and their human counterparts. The contaminated animals were required to be slaughtered and were buried in pits. Whether PBBs are leaking from the pits or not, no one can be certain. We know little of the ultimate fate of the products containing PBBs, since disposed of, or still in use. This type of flame retardant is still in use: PBBs and brominated diphenyl ethers are now found in measurable quantities in Atlantic cod, sperm whales, seals, dolphins, and other marine animals.[45-47]

Before PBB production was stopped in November 1974, the company produced 6.2 million pounds of Firemaster. This was a chemically stable product, intended to be incorporated into plastic products such as housings for business machines, radios, televisions, thermostats, shavers, hand tools, and miscellaneous small automotive parts. We know nothing of the workers

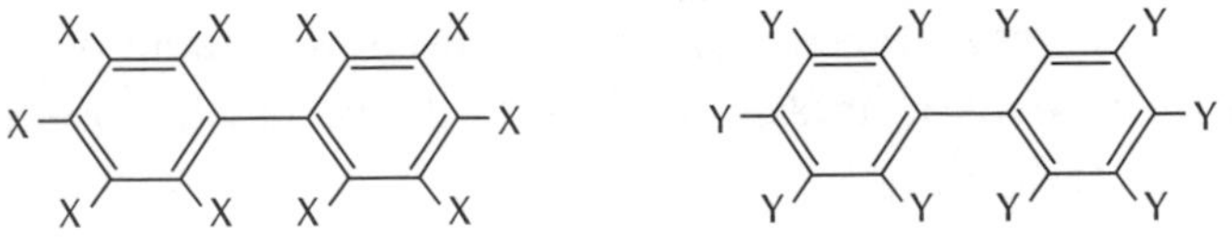

PCB — polychlorinated biphenyl   PBB — polybrominated biphenyl
X = chlorine or hydrogen (1 to 10)   Y = bromine or hydrogen (1 to 10)

Figure 8.4
Chemical structure of halogenated bi-phenyls

who manufactured those products, but we have learned that a dioxin form of PBBs, polybrominated dibenzo-*p*-dioxins, has been measured in the fat of a young man whose exposure to PBBs had come from a television set as he played computer games in a small enclosed room some 13 years earlier.[48]

PBBs have powerful adverse effects upon the thyroid, the immune, vascular, and nervous systems, are toxic to the unborn, and are carcinogenic.[49] I reported two cases of PBB-associated cancer in humans; the first in 1988,[50] involving the colon, the second in 1991, involving the stomach and esophagus.[51] We do know that PBBs are found in the milk of animals and humans, but we do not know how and if PBBs are contributing to breast cancer.

POLYCHLORINATED BIPHENYLS

Polychlorinated biphenyls (PCBs) provide a story of contamination second to none. PCBs were manufactured solely by Monsanto Chemical Corporation at its plants in Sauget, Illinois, just east of St. Louis, Missouri, and in Anniston, Alabama. PCBs were sold to various companies and were marketed under a number of trade names and incorporated into a myriad of products.

Names and corporations included Arochlor (Monsanto); Clophen, Fenclor, Inerteen (Westinghouse); Kanechlor, Phenoclor, Pyralene, Pyranol (General Electric); and Santotherm and Therminol (Monsanto).

Because of relative resistance to fire, PCBs were used as coolants in electrical transformers and capacitors. Such equipment included large electrical power systems of locomotives and generating plants, as well as smaller devices, such as electric utility equipment, air conditioners, and ballasts that run the fluorescent lights in homes and offices. By 1976 17 United States capacitor manufacturers were using PCBs at 19 sites, and 13 transformer manufacturers operated at 18 different sites.[52]

PCBs had other desirable properties: they were chemically stable, resistant to break-down, and relatively inexpensive. PCBs were incorporated into hydraulic and heat transfer systems, gas turbines, vacuum pumps, adhesives, plasticizers, textiles surface coatings, sealants, paints, printing inks, and carbonless carbon paper.[53]

Monsanto's Manager of Environmental Control wrote in 1970: "There is ample evidence from many laboratories that certain species of birds which are at the top of the marine food chain cannot reproduce properly when PCBs are present in their diets."[54] Later that year he expressed interest in the presence of dibenzofuran in the Arochlor manufacturing process, urging the Alabama Monsanto plant to determine the source of contamination.[55] Despite this documentation, Monsanto has steadfastly denied the presence of these contaminants.[56]

Beginning in 1971, Monsanto voluntarily restricted domestic sales of PCBs for transformers and capacitors, requiring them to be used only in closed systems. As a result, production decreased to about 50% from the peak years before the mid 1970s, but still amounted to about 40 million pounds a year. Considering the permanence of PCBs in the environment, and their hormonal effects, the total amount from all sources is staggering. Production of PCBs began in 1929, and by 1976, EPA estimated that 1.4 billion pounds had been produced; 150 million pounds exported, 750 million pounds in service, 500 million pounds having entered the environment, 300 million pounds in landfills, 150 million pounds in air, water, soil, and sediments; and 50 million pounds degraded or incinerated.[57] When EPA's numbers are added together, the sum is 1.9 billion pounds of PCBs, leaving a half million pounds unaccounted for.

Bloomington is noted not only for its world-famous music school at Indiana University, but for having the nation's largest volume of environmental PCBs. Since 1957, this city was home to Westinghouse's capacitor plant. Considering the problem of PCBs in the Bloomington area, the Agency for Toxic Substances and Disease Registry (ATSDR) convened a battery of in-house personnel and outside experts to "assess any public health implications of incinerating polychlorinated biphenyls (PCB)-contaminated waste associated with six hazardous waste sites in the area."[58]

Before addressing the panel's findings, it may be useful to think about the language in the document. What does "any public health implications" mean? Given the toxicology, persistence, and spread of PCBs, hardly a person exists worldwide who hasn't been contaminated with PCBs, and contamination is a virtual certainty in Bloomington.

Language has a way of obscuring reality, and choice of language may obscure the reality of PCB contamination in Bloomington. What are the "health" implications? Is *Brave New World* now here? These are *sickness* implications. Let us understand that the national debate on "Health Care" is in truth, *sickness* care. When we say she "lost" her breast to cancer, we're sanitizing the truth. Her breast was *amputated*. We're not addressing *health*, we're addressing *sickness*.

"Health Effects" conclusions of the Executive Summary of the ATSDR document number eight in all. Four conclusions include as wording "new research," "more research," "further research, and "further study." A fifth notes "qualitative exposure analysis . . . is needed." And so it appears taxpayers' money, time, and effort have been expended to waffle on a public *sickness* issue, and Bloomington is not an isolated situation.

The panel deserves credit for noting various adverse effects due to PCB exposure, including: carcinogenic, reproductive, developmental, neurologic, immunologic, and adverse effects to the skin, liver, cardiovascular, and endocrine/thyroid systems. But what to do about the PCBs and their adverse effects remains another problem. While the panel largely addressed the feasibility and problems of PCB-waste incineration, it noted "some people argue that we should not employ these technologies, and the wastes should be stored in concrete bunkers until a safe technology that won't affect public health is developed."[59]

The plan proposed for Bloomington to build an incinerator to "dispose" of the PCBs from contaminated soils has been blocked by continuing community opposition. Westinghouse documents claim that "revenues from the operation of the incinerator are expected to partially offset the Corporations' [Westinghouse] clean-up costs," . . . and "management continues to believe that the ultimate aggregate cost of environmental remediation by the Corporation will not result in a material adverse effect on its future financial condition or results of operations."[60]

Unmentioned in the ATSRD report, however, is the fact that this one city is the repository for 650 million cubic yards of PCB-contaminated soil. And this is just one area. What are the cumulative amounts of contamination worldwide? Can we expect that Monsanto's PCBs and its public-*sickness* implications will be with us for generations?

Nowhere in the Bloomington report is the suggestion that the manufacturer who profited by PCB production should pay for the cleanup. Some believe that a portion of Monsanto's profits from sales of Nutrasweet, bovine growth hormone, its pesticide Roundup, its Roundup-ready genetically engineered agricultural soybean and other plant products, and pharmaceuticals from its Searle[61] division could be diverted to these ends.

History is once again a teacher, one we have not heeded. Studies in the 1930s showed a myriad of medical problems in people exposed to PCBs. These included liver damage, a skin condition called chloracne, neurological and immunological damage, tumors, and damage to the adrenal glands. The study by Dr. Falk and his associates, cited earlier, found elevated PCBs levels along with DDT in the women with breast cancer. PCBs behave as estrogens, can pass the placenta into the developing baby, and are concentrated in breast milk. Given a 10- to 20-year latency for cancer to develop, contamination at various sites may have contributed to the escalating breast cancer incidence, but testing specific to these sites has not been done.

And studies; studies by whom and supported by which corporation? When one read the statement: "There are few animal data that support the carcinogenicity and health effects of lower-chlorinated PCB mixtures. This data gap may be addressed by a study being conducted by General Electric that is expected to be completed by the end of 1995" to attorney David McCrea of Bloomington, who represents PCB-exposed persons, he replied "that's asking the rapist to baby-sit."

How can one trust PCB animal tests, conducted by a corporation whose attorneys argue in court against the validity of animal tests? In at least one case, involving General Electric, this delaying tactic was ruled against by a federal appeals court.[62]

From the 1930s through the end of the 1970s, Westinghouse and General Electric were the biggest purchasers of PCBs. Because of PCB pollution problems, both have become defendants in legal cases, spreading from the Hudson River to the Paoli railroad yard near Philadelphia. General Electric is listed as a "PRP" (potentially responsible party) at 51 Superfund sites located from coast to coast,[63] and yet, in 1991, GE admitted spending only "approximately $125 million on remedial cleanups and related studies." That $125 million dedicated to cleanup based upon revenues of $60,236 million calculates to but 0.2% of corporate income.

GE operated the Hanford Nuclear Reservation for two decades, beginning in 1946, leaving behind nuclear and chemical contamination. Among its products, GE makes aircraft engines, appliances, industrial generators, plastic and medical equipment. It is the owner of NBC-TV, and Westinghouse bought CBS. The public may well wonder if and when reporters from either network will be allowed to address chemical and nuclear pollution issues.

A GE x-ray machine may diagnose our cancer, GE magnetic resonant or ultrasound equipment may find our metastases, and GE-powered x-ray equipment may radiate our cancerous bodies, perhaps caused by GE's chemical and nuclear releases. And during the while, we may watch television, owned by the same company.

At the very least, each woman diagnosed with breast cancer deserves an assay of her fat for the chemical invaders: PCBs, chlordane/heptachlor, dioxins, and DDT and its kin. These are the biological markers reflective of past exposure. Such tests are not routinely ordered by physicians, and are often not covered by medical insurance. But who is more able to pay for these tests than the corporation that bragged: "Monsanto is a party to a number of lawsuits and claims, which it is vigorously defending. . . . Certain of these actions seek damages in very large amounts. While the results of litigation cannot be predicted with certainty, management believes, based upon the advice of Company counsel, that the final outcome of such litigation will not have a material adverse effect on Monsanto's consolidated financial position."[65]

How has the lack of restraint by corporation interests escaped our notice? How many people read the fine print in corporate annual reports? Who pays attention to Boards of Directors, peopled with ex-military, ex-EPA officials, and presidents of universities, often recipients of corporate research funds? Who then pays for this egregious contamination? With loss of health? Loss of job and family? Loss of life?

Added to chemicals known to cause cancer are chemicals that disrupt the endocrine systems in women, men, children, and the unborn. While the list is not extensive, so far, hormonal testing should be required of all persistent chemicals of related structure. The EPA has held a number of meetings to address hormone disruption testing; however, nothing concrete has been decided as of this writing. How many more endocrine-disrupting chemicals remain undetected is anybody's guess.

A CALL FOR A BAN ON CHLORINE-BASED ORGANIC PRODUCTS

Chlorine is undeniably one of the building blocks of life, an essential part of nutrition, of life itself. But with all too many basic chemicals, chlorine has been corrupted by the creativity of technology and the marketplace and used to produce and sell inappropriate and dangerous products. While some chlorine-containing products are essential to medicine, commerce, and public health, far too many are cosmetic, in the worse sense of the word. Few have been injured by common lawn weeds, yet millions of dollars have been spent on "lawn care" pesticides that serve no useful purpose other than to create a lawn of uniform grass. Pesticides, plastics, including vinyl chloride, and industrial solvents account for about 80% of all chlorine use.[66] Many are clearly not essential.

The "birth-to-death" cycle of chlorine use has many holes through which chlorinated chemicals leave the cycle and enter the world's environment. Chlorinated chemicals leak out during production, use, disposal, and incineration of each product, be it from pesticides, plastic wrap, industrial paints and solvents, pulp and paper bleaching, or incineration of any of the above.

Foods and merchandise could be better packaged and sold in glass containers, rather than in chlorine-containing plastics. Omitting plastic objects from the waste stream removes them as a source of dioxins in incinerators.

Paper bleached by chlorine has become a source of dioxin contamination. Do we really need bleached paper on which to print our newspapers and other reading materials, or to make our coffee filters and toilet tissue?

The EPA's various statutes, especially those regulated under the pesticide and toxic substances laws, are extremely difficult to change, and products are not required to be proved harmless prior to marketing. Adverse effects include not only cancer, but harm to the neurological, immunological, endocrine, and reproductive systems, and harm to the unborn. Opting for a change in practice, if not a change in the law, unless these chemicals of concern can be proved to be safe, it would be prudent to avoid use and exposure to at least the following chemicals, chlorinated and all pesticides:[67]

Alachlor
Atrazine
Benzene hexachloride
Chlordane and oxychlordane
DDT, DDE, and DDD
DBCP (dibromochloropropane)—soil fumigant
2,4-D dichlorophenoxy acetic acid ⎫
2,4,5-T trichlorophenoxy acetic acid ⎭ "AGENT ORANGE"
Dicofol
Dieldrin
Endosulfan
Heptachlor and its epoxide
Hexachlorobenzene
Lindane
Mirex

Nitrofen
Pentachlorophenol (wood preservative and herbicide)
Toxaphene

INCINERATION—A SOURCE
OF CARCINOGENS

Of particular concern in cancer causation is the release from incinerators of dioxins, dibenzofurans, and PCBs. A call to halt construction of new incinerators has been made. So too is the call to require those under operation to trap and contain all emissions and ash. More to the point is a need to stop incineration that produces emissions contaminated with dioxins, dibenzofurans, heavy metals, and radioisotopes and to educate the public to decrease waste.

Incineration has become an increasingly popular technology to deal with our mountain of garbage and unwanted by-products of production. Unfortunately, out of sight has not become out of mind, nor out of body. Burning of chlorine-containing articles, be they municipal household wastes or medical wastes, generates many combustion products. These chemicals leave the smokestack, are carried by wind and rain, where they attract radioactive particles released from bomb testing and nuclear reactors, fall to earth and become deposited upon plants, soil, and water. Plants absorb the contaminants, and these in turn are fed to cattle, sheep, and poultry, thus entering the human food chain. Fish, a major food source for many, have become contaminated, notably in the Great Lakes, the Salton Sea, even from the deep ocean.[68,69] Dioxins, furans, and PCBs become more concentrated with each pass along the food chain, causing damage to the endocrine systems of animals along the way, winding up in the bodies of ourselves and our babies.

None of these changes will be easy. The movement by transnational corporations, abetted by compliant business-oriented governments has been well documented in Fagan and Lavelle's *Toxic Deception—How the Chemical Industry Manipulates Science, Bends the Law, and Endangers Your Health,*[70] and in Korten's *When Corporations Rule the World.*[71] Entrenchment of economic forces, powerful political and public relations allies, and the antiregulatory stance of the current U.S. Congress will in all likelihood impede, if not halt, attempts at reform. This is most likely to occur unless there is a groundswell of cancer patients, their families and supporters who say "no more business as usual." We want, we demand, and we have a right to prevent cancer!

REFERENCES

1. Wargo, J. Our Children's toxic Legacy—How Science and Law Fail to Protect Us from Pesticides. Yale University Press. New Haven CT. pp. 15–42. 1996.

2. Mrak, E. M. Chairman. Report of the Secretary's Commission on Pesticides and Their Relationship to Environmental Health. U.S. Dept. Health, Education and Welfare. pp. 7–19, and text. 1969.

3. Perthane, also marketed by Rhom and Haas has been discontinued as of 1994. Farm Chemical Handbook.

4. Kelce, W. R., Stone, C. R., Laws, S. C., Gray, L. E., Kemppainen, J. A., Wilson, E. M. The persistent DDT metabolite p, p´DDE is a potent androgen receptor antagonist. Nature. 1995.

5. Wassermann, M., Norgueira, D. P., Tomatis, L., Mirra, A. P., Shibata, H., Arie, G., Cucos, S., Wassermann, D. Organochlorine compounds in neoplastic and adjacent apparently normal breast tissue. Bull. Environ. Contam. Toxicol. 15(4): 478–484, 1976.

6. Falck, F., Jr., Ricci, A., Jr., Wolff, M. S., Gobold, J., Deckers, P. Pesticides and polychlorinated biphenyl residues in human breast lipids and their relation to breast cancer. Arch. Environ. Health. 47(2): 143–146, 1992.

7. Wolff, M. S., Toniolo, P. G., Lee, E. W., Rivera, M., Dubin, N. Blood levels of organochlorine residues and risk of breast cancer. J. Nat. Cancer Inst. 85: 648–652, 1993.

8. Krieger, N., Wolff, M. S., Hiatt, R. A., Rivera, M., Vogelman, J., Orentreuch, N. Breast cancer and serum organochlorines: a prospective study among white, black and Asian women. J. Nat. Cancer Inst. 86: 589–599, 1994.

9. Hunter, D. J., Hankinson, S. E., Laden, F., Colditz, G. A., Manson, J. E., Willett, W. C., Speizer, F. E., Wolff, M. S. Plasma organochlorine levels and the risk of breast cancer. New Engl. J. Med. 337(18): 1253–1258, 1997.

10. Rachel's Environment and Health Weekly. #574. Montague, P. Ed. 1997.

11. Safe, S. H. Editorial: Xenoestrogens and breast cancer. New Engl. J. Med. 337(18): 1303–1304, 1997.

12. Ibid.

13. vom Saal, F. S., Welshons, W. V., Hansen, L. G. Organochlorine residues and breast cancer. New Engl. J. Med. 338(14), 988, 1998.

14. Kelce, W. R., Stone, C. R., Laws, S. C., Gray, L. E., Kemppainen, J. A., Wilson, E. M. Persistent DDT metabolic p, p´-DDE is a potent androgen receptor antagonist. Nature. 375: 581–585, 1995.

15. Kolata, G. DDT and breast cancer. New York Times. p. 26. October 30, 1997.

16. Rachel's Environment and Health Weekly. #572. Montague, P., Ed. 1997.

17. Hayes, W. J., Jr. Pesticides Studied in Man. Williams & Wilkins, Baltimore. p. 187. 1982.

18. Ibid., p. 190.

19. Hsieh, C. C., Tzonou, A., Trichopoulos, D. Birth order and breast cancer risk. Cancer Causes Control. 2: 95–98, 1991.

20. Toth, B. A critical review of experiments in chemical carcinogenesis using newborn animals. Cancer Res. 28: 727–738, 1968.

21. Kutz, F. W., Yobs, A. R., Strassman, S. C. Racial stratification of organochlorine insecticide residues in human adipose tissue. J. Occup. Med. 19(9): 619–622, 1977.

22. Strassman, S. C. EPA National Human Monitoring Program. Letter to US Congressman R. Dellums. 2 pages. July 20, 1979.

23. Davies, J., Edmundson, W. F., Rattonelli, A. The role of social class in human pesticide pollution. Amer. J. Epidemiol. 96: 334–341, 1972.

24. Marquardt, S. Greenpeace. Personal communication. September. 1994.

25. MacGregor, J. S. Changes in the amount and proportion of DDT and its metabolites, DDE and DDD, in the marine environment off southern California, 1949–1972. Fishery Bull. 72: 275–293, 1974.

26. Rashad, M. N., Klemmer, H. W. Association between serum cholesterol and serum organochlorine residues. Bull. Environ. Contam. Toxicol. 15(4): 475–477, 1976.   ·

27. EPA, Health Assessment Document for 2,3,7,8-tetrachlorodibenzo-p-dioxin: Vol. I and II; Estimating Exposure to Dioxin-Like Compounds, Vol. I, II, and III. 1994.

28. Burrows, B. A., Chalmers, T. C. Cesium-137/potassium-40 rations in firewood ashes as a reflection of worldwide radioactive contamination of the environment. In: Trends in Cancer Mortality in Industrial Countries. Davis, D. L., Hoel, D., Eds. New York Acad. Sci. 609: 334–337, 1990.

29. Connett, E., Connett, P., Eds. Waste Not. No. 300. September, 1994. 82 Judson St., Canton, NY 13617. Phone 315-379-9200.

30. U.S. v. Vertac Chemical Corp., E. D. Ark. No. LR-C-80-109. 10/23/98.

31. Bureau of National Affairs. Hercules, Uniroyal found liable for $102 million at Vertac Superfund site. Toxics Law Reporter. 12(22): 700, 1998.

32. Chaloupka, K., Krishnan, V., Safe, S. Polynuclear aromatic hydrocarbon carcinogens as antiestrogens in MCF-7 human breast cancer cells: role of the Ah receptor. Carcinogenesis. 13(12) 2233–2239, 1992.

33. Other trade names include: G-11, AT-7, Bilevon, Dermadex, Exofene, Gamophen, Hexosan, Surgi-Cen, and Surofene.

34. Baughman, R., Newton, L. Analysis for tetrachlorodibenzo-p-dioxins in a French talcum powder—hexachlorophene formulation implicated in the death of a number of infants. Monograph. Department of Chemistry, Harvard University. 6 pages. October 1972.

35. Fingerhut, M. A., Halperin, W. E., Marlow, D. A, Piacitelli, L. A., Honchar, P. A., Sweeney, M. H., Greife, A. L., Dill, P. A., Steenland, K. Suruda, A. J. Cancer mortality in workers exposed to 2,3,7,8-tetrachlorodibenzo-p-dioxin. New Engl. J. Med. 324:212–218, 1991.

36. Egeland, G. M., Sweeney, M. H., Fingerhut, M. A., Wille, K. K., Schnorr, T. M., Halperin, W. E. Total serum testosterone and gonadotropins in workers exposed to dioxins. Amer. J. Epidemiol. 139(3): 272–281, 1994.

37. Safe, S., Astroff, B., Harris, M., Zacharewski, T. 2,3,7,8-tetrachlorodebenzo-p-

dioxin (TCDD) and its related compounds as antiestrogens: characterization and mechanism of action. Pharmacol. Toxicol. 69(6): 400–409, 1991.

38. U.S. Patents No. 3,244,586, April 5, 1966, No. 3,326,752, June 20, 1967.

39. U.S. EPA, Registration Standard (Second Round Review) for the Reregistration of Pesticide Products Containing Chlorpyrifos. p. 42. June 1989.

40. Barber, D. T. Dow Chemical Co. Letter to Edwards, D., EPA, Re: Potential formation of a dioxino product during the synthesis of Dursban-F. 5 pages. September 24, 1987; plus Appendix B consisting of 1 page; and Analytical Method, 6 pages, dated March 25, 1986.

41. Marquardt, S. Greenpeace. Personal communication. 9-13-94.

42. Mussalo-Rauhamaa, H., Hasanen, E., Pyysalo, H., Antervo, K., Kauppila, R., Pantzar, P. Occurrence of beta-hexachlorocyclohexane in breast cancer patients. Cancer. 66(10): 2124–2128, 1990.

43. Dusuch, K. Sigurson, E., Hall, W. N., Dean, A. G. Cancer rates in a community exposed to low levels of creosote components in municipal water. Minn. Med. 63: 803–806, 1980.

44. Lee, S. D., Grant, L., Eds. Health and ecological assessment of polycyclic aromatic hydrocarbons. J. Environ. Pathol. Toxicol. 5(1): 250–251, 1981.

45. Pijenberg, A. M. C. M., Everts, J. W., de Boer, J., Boon, J. P. Polybrominated biphenyl and diphenyl flame retardants: Analysis, toxicity, and environmental occurrence. Rev. Environ. Contam. Toxicol. 141: 2–25, 1995.

46. de Boer, J. Organochlorine compounds and bromodiphenylethers in livers of Atlantic cod (Gadus morhua) from the North Sea, 1977–1987. Chemosphere. 18(11/12): 2131–2140, 1989.

47. de Boer, J., Wester, P. G., Klanier, H. J. C., Lewis, W. E., Boon, J. P. Do flame retardants threaten ocean life? Nature. 394:27–28, 1994.

48. de Boer, J., Robertson, L. W., Dettmer, F., Wichmann, H., Bahadir, M. Polybrominated diphenyethers in human adipose tissue and relation with watching television—a case study. Correspondence from DLO-Netherlands Institute for Fisheries Research. IJmuiden, The Netherlands.

49. Sherman, J. D., Polybrominated biphenyl exposure and human cancer: report of a case and public health implications. Toxicol. Indust. Health. 7(3): 197—205, 1991.

50. Sherman, J. D. Chemical Exposure and Disease. Princeton Scientific Publishing Co., Inc. Princeton, NJ. pp. 126–127, 1994.

51. Sherman. Op. cit. 1991.

52. Farlee, C. PCB residues in humans: Is there evidence of differential impact on racial minorities? EPA. pp. 69, 89. August 9, 1979.

53. NCR was one manufacturer of carbonless carbon paper, according to Business Week. pp. 69–71. August 12, 1991.

54. Pappageorge, W. B., Monsanto Co., letter to Jenkins, F., Sprague Electric Co. of North Adams, MA. 3 pages. July 8, 1970.

55. Pappageorge, W. B. Memo to Savage, J. R. 1 page. October 26, 1970.

56. Coppolino, E. C. Pandora's poison. Sierra Magazine. 41–45, 74–77. September/October 1994.

57. Federal Register. 41(64): 14134–14136, April 1, 1976.

58. Lichtveld, M. Y., Susten, A, S. Proceedings of the expert panel workshop to evaluate the public health implications of the treatment and disposal of polychlorinated biphenyls-contaminated waste. ATSDR, HHS, USPHS. 1994

59. Ibid., pp. 3–36.

60. Westinghouse Annual Report. p.19. 1992.

61. The connection between chemicals that cause sickness and those prescribed to those sick is amply demonstrated by Monsanto's Searle division: Aldactazide, Aldactone, Aminophylline, Calan, Cytotec, Demulen, Dramamine, Envoid, Flagyl, Kerlone, Lomotil, Nitrodisc, Norpace, and Theo-24, products used to control blood pressure, relieve asthma, for birth control, to stop diarrhea, and a nonsteroidal anti-inflammatory drug that causes abortion.

62. United States Court of Appeals for the Third Circuit. No. 92-1995. In re: Paoli Railroad Yard PCB Litigation. Files August 31, 1994.

63. INFACT. Bringing GE to Light: General Electric's Trail of Radioactive and Toxic contamination form the Company's Nuclear Weapons Work. P. O. Box 3223, South Pasadena, CA 91031. October 1990.

64. INFACT's film about GE, "Deadly Deception," was nominated for an Academy Award.

65. General Electric Annual Report. p. 42. 1991. Reduced to $120 million for 1992.

66. Monsanto Annual Report. p. 49. 1991.

67. Thornton, J. Chlorine, Human Health and the Environment—The Breast Cancer Warning. Greenpeace. 67 pages. October 1993. (This may be ordered from Greenpeace, 1436 U Street, N.W., Washington, D.C. 20009.)

68. Thornton. Op cit.

69. Elder, D. L., Fowler, S. W. Polychlorinated biphenyls: Penetration into the deep ocean by zooplankton fecal pellet transport. Science. 197: 459–461, 1977.

70. Eisenreich, S. J., Looney, B. B., Thornton, J. D. Airborne organic contaminants in the Great Lakes ecosystem. Environ. Sci. Technol. 15(1): 30–38, 1981.

71. Fagan, D., Lavelle, M. Toxic Deception—How the Chemical Industry Manipulates Science, Bends the Law, and Endangers Your Health. Birch Lane Press, Carol Publishing Group. Secaucus, NJ. 294 pages. 1996.

72. Korten, D. When Corporations Rule the World. Kumarian Press, Berrett-Koehler Publishers. West Hartford, CT. 374 pages. 1995.

9

TAMOXIFEN
CHEMICAL MANIPULATION

First do not harm.
—Hippocrates

In 1995, public hearings were held in California,[1] following which tamoxifen was designated as a carcinogen by the state of California.[2] Substantiating the finding is a 16-page list of articles and comments, relied upon by that state's Carcinogen Identification Committee, available from the California state offices in Sacramento.[3] How did this proven carcinogen become the drug of choice for treating breast cancer, and for the "prevention" of breast cancer?

The media hype following the National Cancer Institute announcement that tamoxifen prevents breast cancer bears some scrutiny.[4]

It sounds good, but is it really? Tamoxifen has been promoted to two groups of women: those already diagnosed as having breast cancer and those "at risk" to develop the disease. The first option proposed for *prevention* of breast cancer is a drug: tamoxifen; a second "option" is *prophylactic* bilateral mastectomy. The latter is hardly an option, and the first is not without harm. Neither addresses the issue of causation and primary prevention.

WOMEN WHO HAVE BREAST CANCER

A woman who has breast cancer is put in the unenviable position of having to decide which of the treatment regimes she is willing to undergo in order to achieve arrest of her disease. When it comes to therapeutic agents for which there are serious side effects and controversy concerning efficacy, the problem becomes very difficult. One decision the breast cancer patient may have to make is whether she ought to take tamoxifen or not. Cancer is a serious disease, and most of us will do just about anything to put malignancy at bay. There are studies crediting tamoxifen use with prolonging survival and decreasing reoccurrence of cancer in the affected as well as the other breast. The 1987 collaborative treatment trial, utilizing multiple therapies, including tamoxifen showed a 9.2% better disease-free state and survival in the first 5 years.[5] Unfortunately, after 5 years, these improvements did not persist.[6] But this was not a revelation: in two earlier studies, only about 30% of women treated with tamoxifen had a complete or partial remission that lasted for a year or more.[7,8]

Even the current NCI press release admitted that use of tamoxifen for more than 5 years showed no improvement, and "showed a trend toward more adverse effects." Hormonal manipulation for breast cancer is not new, only different. Previously, surgical removal of a woman's ovaries was the method of choice to block a woman's own hormones. And when oophorectomy was not successful, a woman's pituitary was removed surgically or destroyed by radiation. It was this procedure, ablation of her pituitary by implanted radioactive yttrium, that Rachel Carson underwent, shortly before her death.[9] Like others who underwent these procedures, the results were often either not effective or incapacitating, or both.

Still, some combinations of therapy (both hormonal and chemotherapy) appear to prolong survival, used in combination with surgery and radiation. The questions are: which of the 16 or so chemotherapeutic agents, in which combinations, and at what times will improve our chances of survival?

Between 1970 and 1987, more than 3 million women were administered tamoxifen for a cumulative time of more than 5.8 million patient years.[10] Unfortunately, except for specific clinical trials, few records have been kept on women given the drug for therapy.

A review of some 14 different clinical trials in which tamoxifen was given to women with breast cancer showed worrisome results. Although an increased disease-free state was shown in all the trials, the overall survival was improved in but four of the trials, with women older than 50 years achieving the most benefit.[11]

TAMOXIFEN AND BREAST CANCER "PREVENTION"

For this chapter, however, the issue is not only which treatment regime to follow, but whether to participate in an experiment, one touted as a breast cancer prevention trial. The story is interesting, if not especially comforting.

The name tamoxifen achieved widespread publicity in April of 1994. At that time, physicians across the United States received what is known as a "Dear Doctor" letter from Zeneca Corporation, concerning the development of uterine cancer in women receiving tamoxifen, as reported in a large Swedish study.[12] A similar study undertaken in the Netherlands reported a statistically significant excess of uterine cancer in the women after taking tamoxifen for 2 to 5 years, correlated with both cumulative dose and duration of use.[13] These two studies were echoed by a Danish/British study that "detected endometrial abnormalities at various times from the first tablet of tamoxifen."[14]

At the same time as the Zeneca letter went out to physicians, a similar communique, the "Dear Patient" letter, was sent to women participating in the National Surgical Adjuvant Breast and Bowel Project (NSABP), the coordinating center for the tamoxifen breast cancer prevention trial, telling them the same thing. But women patients, taking tamoxifen for treatment of their breast malignancies, not in the official NCI/NSABP trial, received no such warning.

The Breast Cancer Prevention Trial has enrolled women as human guinea pigs to test tamoxifen as a "prevention" against breast cancer. The trial, planned since 1990 and launched in April 1992, enrolled 11,000 women, aiming optimally to enroll 16,000 *healthy* women, between the ages of 35 and 78. The trial closed enrollment in September 1997, at which time, 13,388 women ages 35 and older were enrolled. Half of the women received tamoxifen and half a nonhormonal placebo. A similar proposal to be carried out in England as of 1994 was declined by Britain's Medical Research Council.[15]

In 1995, researchers at Washington University Medical School in St. Louis, Missouri, and the Medical School at Dartmouth calculated that for a 50-year-old woman with a risk for breast cancer twice that of an average woman her age, the increase in longevity would be approximately 9 days.[16]

The tamoxifen experiment was to run for a 5-year period, but when the results of the study were released in April of 1998, only 57% of the enrollees had completed four or more years on the study. The study was carried out at more than 300 sites in the United States and Canada and by investigators who have extensive, some, and no experience or training in the proper conduct of clinical trials, plus little oversight by NIH.[17] Prior to the NSABP tamoxifen investigation, clinical studies under the aegis of NSABP had been carried out at 400 collaborating clinical centers in the United States and Canada; a formidable task to achieve any degree of uniformity, accuracy, and objectivity.

Women were recruited from those at high "risk." Risk was defined as women with a family history of breast cancer—a mother, sister, or other close relative. Family history was advanced as a major risk of developing the disease, ignoring other causes of breast cancer. Women older than 60 were included on the basis of age alone. The NCI press release stated: "The risk of developing breast cancer increases with age, so breast cancer occurs more commonly in women over 60 years of age."[18]

One can't argue with the issue that cancer is commoner in older persons than in younger ones, but isn't one of the reasons for more cancer that the older person has not only lived more years, but during those years has been exposed to carcinogenic agents for a longer period of time? Enrolling the over-60 women, without any other risk factor, also ignores the increase in breast cancer among younger women.

Relying on family history for selection is a significant issue. As evidence emerges, the poisoned environment is clearly playing an overwhelming role in the increase in breast and other cancers. Little considered is the fact that breast cancer, indeed all cancers in families, may be not of genetic cause, but the result of common exposure to radiation, carcinogenic, and hormone-disrupting chemicals. After all, environment is shared within families: neighborhood, housing, food, recreation, etc.

Women were enrolled in the study if they had stopped taking either oral contraceptives or hormone replacement drugs for three months. What effect did the use of these hormonal drugs have on the outcome of the trial? Such questions as duration of use of either or both, level of hormone in the preparation, and exposure to other hormones such as in the diet of those who eat meat appear not to be part of the analysis.

Despite the current alarming statistic that one in eight women in the United States, and one in ten in Canada, will develop breast cancer, it is necessary to understand that seven out of eight United States women will not develop cancer! Until connections to the environment *and* family history *and* breast cancer are fully investigated, the question remains: Is it ethical to give a carcinogenic chemical to seven women (as in seven-out-of-eight) who might never develop breast cancer in the first place?

DEVELOPMENT OF TAMOXIFEN

Tamoxifen was developed by London-based Imperial Chemical Industries (ICI), one of the world's largest and most successful multinational chemical corporations. Tamoxifen is dispensed as a small white tablet, displaying an impression of a woman's head on one side.

Chemically, tamoxifen is a member of the stilbene or substituted-diethylene family, differing little from its chemical cousins diethylstilbestrol (DES) and clomiphene, known to be structurally related by ICI scientists.[19] Its structural relationship to DES demonstrates a story difficult to put in words. Tamoxifen has three phenyl rings, instead of the two rings found in DES, as noted in Figure 9.1.

The structural relationship of tamoxifen to DES is critical. It was DES that caused genital cancers in the daughters of women who were prescribed DES in a misguided effort to prevent miscarriages. Two decades ago, tamoxifen and the pesticides DDT and methoxychlor were demonstrated to share similar biochemical action.[20] Mounting evidence points to organic chemicals, similar to tamoxifen, that are linked to endocrine disruption and cancer. These include some organochlorine pesticides, PCBs, and dioxins.[21] Other

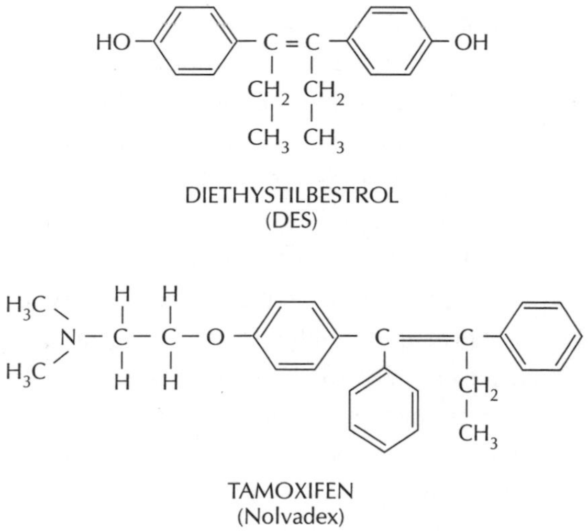

DIETHYSTILBESTROL
(DES)

TAMOXIFEN
(Nolvadex)

Figure 9.1
Chemical structures of DES and tamoxifen.

double-ring chemicals with a single- rather than a double-carbon bond produce adverse effects upon reproduction and hormonal function and demonstrate carcinogenicity.[22-26] These findings have been known for nearly three decades.

The ability of DES to cause cancer was known before tamoxifen was patented and certainly before tamoxifen was developed on a commercial scale.[27-31] Moreover, Zeneca Corporation's Dear Doctor letter stated: "In rodent models of fetal reproductive tract development, tamoxifen ... caused changes in both sexes that are similar to those caused by ... diethylstilbe-strol," reiterating what had been reported previously.[32]

As early as 1967, ICI scientists wrote that "tamoxifen persists for some days in the uterus." In rats, a tamoxifen metabolite was found to influence the translocation of the estrogen receptor to the uterine nucleus. ICI scientists found the antiestrogen action of tamoxifen was related to its ability[33] to bind to estrogen receptors, with "metabolite-B" (more similar in structure to DES), having greater binding ability. Tamoxifen stimulates hypertrophy of the lining of the uterus.[34] In one study, women treated with tamoxifen for over two years had fewer new breast cancers, but an increase in uterine cancer.[35] An Israeli study of 175 post-menopausal breast cancer patients who received continuous tamoxifen therapy found 8.1% developed uterine polyps, 57.2% had atrophic endometrium, and 35.7% had coexisting hyper-plasia of the lining of the uterus.[36]

Not only the use of tamoxifen, but age and hormonal status of a woman may influence the development of uterine cancer. In women who started tamoxifen therapy many years after menopause, there was an estrogenic effect on the uterus, causing endometrial thickening, polyps, and atypical cells. For this reason, patients should be monitored by transvaginal ultra-sound and Doppler imaging to detect early lesions.[37]

The paradoxical estrogenic/antiestrogenic effects may occur because the binding of tamoxifen and its metabolites to the estrogen receptor fails to induce transcriptional activation of all elements in target genes,[38,39] and thus becomes expressed as an estrogen antagonist (antiestrogen) in breast tissue, and estrogen agonist (similar to estrogen) in endometrial tissue.[40]

One-quarter of patients in the United Kingdom breast cancer preven-tion study had atypical endometrial hyperplasia and polyps.[41] Fisher, the director of the United States trial, estimated the risk of endometrial cancer in women taking tamoxifen to be 1 to 2 per 1000 per year[42] Stating the usual risk of so many cancers per 1 million population, the given risk of 1 to

2 per 1000 translates into 1000 to 2000 women with uterine cancer. To whom is this acceptable?

Animal tests shows that tamoxifen had the ability to cause genetic damage in the livers of animals and in the protein extracts of human liver cells.[43,44]

Early development of tamoxifen was as a contraceptive, but it functioned actually as an abortant, preventing implantation of the fetus, analogous to a chemical IUD (intrauterine device), resulting in termination of pregnancy as tested in rats. And it was by no means 100% effective.[45,46] Rats given from 0.3 to 2.4 times the human dose of tamoxifen developed genital changes in both sexes, similar to those caused by estradiol, ethinyl estradiol, and diethylstilbestrol (DES).[47]

Tamoxifen was promoted also to prevent osteoporosis, but that too has been disputed. Patients from a Danish Breast Cancer Cooperative Group were analyzed. Their study suggested "that tamoxifen does not seem to offer protection against fractures in old age and may even increase the risk of fractures at particular sites."[48] The NCI release reported fewer fractures of the hip, wrist, and spine in the group taking tamoxifen.[49] The incidence was 47 versus 71 in those not taking tamoxifen, but there is no information as to the level of activity of each group. It appears premature to attribute this difference as a benefit to using tamoxifen. Athletic active women may have more injuries than sedentary ones, who on the contrary are more likely to develop osteoporosis.

Given that pre-menopausal women taking tamoxifen are urged not to take birth control pills for conception control, the specter of a child with tamoxifen-induced birth defects or post-adolescent development of cancer is a valid concern. Currently, the period of time for the expression of cancer in post-adolescence has not been fully achieved for tamoxifen-exposed offspring. Birth defects are reported in a child delivered of a woman who had taken 20 mg daily of tamoxifen until 20 weeks gestation. The baby girl had clitoral enlargement, a single urethra/vaginal opening, and fused labia.[50] As if the cancer and birth defects associated with tamoxifen use were not of sufficient concern, interference with immunological function has been found in test animals.[51] Considering that an intact and well-functioning immunological system is required to keep malignancy under control, this effect may be of greater significance than we now appreciate.

In pre-menopausal women, with or without breast cancer, administration of tamoxifen resulted in elevated estradiol and prolactin levels, while in post-menopausal breast cancer patients, tamoxifen was without effect.

Prolactin is a hormone normally released by the maternal pituitary gland at the time of birth to allow breast development and milk production for the suckling infant. Abnormal prolactin release has been correlated with a number of chemicals that act as promoters of breast cancer. This issue is discussed in Chapter 8 (Hormones Too).

ICI-supported research continued and showed mixed actions: it had antiestrogenic effects in the rat, while acting as a potent estrogen in the mouse.[52] Tested again in rats, tamoxifen promoted hormone-independent mammary tumors.[53] And, ICI research revealed liver carcinogenicity and both ovarian and testicular tumors in mice.[54]

Some women develop mastalgia, more commonly called painful breasts, often associated with the normal swelling that occurs just prior to menstruation. Other than discomfort, it is not a serious disease, but various drug treatments have been suggested. Promoted in the mid 1980s to treat mastalgia, the author of a clinical study cautioned "administration of tamoxifen to a patient with undiagnosed malignancy could lead to the emergence of an endocrine unresponsive tumor."[55]

WOMEN ADVOCATING FOR WOMEN

Thanks to data collected and analyzed by members of the National Women's Health Network (NWHN),[56] a publically funded advocacy organization, there appears to have been a disregard or at least a glossing over of concerns about the toxicity of tamoxifen by those eager to obtain clinical trials. Network members, even before the clinical trials had begun, documented known risks associated with tamoxifen use: uterine cancer, increased blood clotting, impaired vision, and cataract formation. Unfortunately, there is no data base for women taking tamoxifen outside of the specific trials. There are reports that tamoxifen use is associated with damage to the eyes,[57] including retinopathy,[58] even at low dose and reported as early as 1983.[59]

In organ culture, tamoxifen blocked chloride channels in the lens of the eye. These channels are essential to maintain hydration and transmittance of light through the lens. This adverse effect is totally independent of estrogen receptor binding.[60]

In the spring of 1991, NCI announced that it was going ahead with a tamoxifen breast cancer "prevention" trial. NWHN representatives testified before FDA officials in an effort to persuade them to amend the protocol and address the hazards that had been observed. Three women testified on behalf of the network and stated specifically: "1) There are no data on the safety of long-term use of tamoxifen in humans, 2) the animal data are not comforting, 3) public health interventions should be health-promoting or at least non-toxic."[61] That the testimony came from eminently qualified women, one a physician and a second who held a Ph. D. , did little to stop the FDA.

Following the April 1998 NCI press releases, the NWHN remained "cautiously optimistic that tamoxifen may benefit women with the BRCA gene and other women at high risk of developing cancer. For women without an elevated risk of breast cancer, the benefits of tamoxifen remain very questionable."[62] Whether the women who developed cancer tested positive for the breast cancer gene or not is unknown. It was not a part of the study protocol. The NWHN recommend regular exercise, and eating a low-fat, high-fiber diet rich in cruciferous vegetables, which not only may be preventive, but carries no risk of adverse effects.

When the "prevention trial" consent form came out in January 1992, the most up-to-date information concerning uterine cancer in humans was not included. This omission gave women the impression that risks were low. Risk of developing life-threatening blood clots were unreported, and liver cancer, produced in rodents, was misrepresented.

By June 1992, barely 2 months after the trials had started, more information emerged about liver damage in women taking tamoxifen. Later that summer, researchers published data showing eye damage in tamoxifen users.[63]

During the summer and fall of that year, the network cooperated with a Congressional committee as to problems with the adequacy of the consent form used in the trials. This investigation revealed that 68% of the forms either omitted or altered one or more key points from the NCI-approved model form. Some of the forms did not meet minimum legal requirements for informed consent.

By October 1992, the findings were presented to then Director of NIH, Dr. Bernadine Healey, who defended the trial. But, by early 1993, reports emerged that women taking tamoxifen had developed endometrial and gastrointestinal cancers. In January 1994, reporters found that Dr. Fisher, based at the University of Pittsburgh and heading the project, had been aware of new endometrial cancers in breast cancer patients, and that several women had died as a result of these new cancers.

One logical question is: Why weren't regular and comprehensive gyneco-logical examinations a required part of the NCI protocol from the start, given that 23 women had developed uterine cancer in an earlier "B-14" tamoxifen study, managed by the same group (NSABP) that oversaw the NCI study?[64] In the face of the human and animal findings, it is difficult to understand the rationale behind reluctance to recommend regular gynecological examina-tion of women taking tamoxifen.[65]

It is essential to understand that there is no official gynecological exami-nation program in effect for women with breast cancer being *treated* with tamoxifen, as contrasted with those participating in the official study. Likewise, there is no nationwide program to assemble and maintain records on women prescribed tamoxifen for *treatment* of breast cancer.

Using data from the B-14 program that had demonstrated an increased endometrial cancer rate of 1.6/1000 in tamoxifen-treated women, it can be calculated that 8 times that, or 12.8 additional women, can be expected to develop gynecological cancer among the 8000 women treated with tamoxifen. Is that hazard acceptable? Is the trial ethical, given that the original protocol neither specified nor provided funding for gynecological examinations? Merely reporting vaginal bleeding to ones' physician is insufficient: uterine malignancy may develop in the absence of overt bleeding.

As of 1992, the NSABP Consent Form to be agreed to by women taking part in the trial stated: "Other medications and all physicians' or hospital costs will be charged to me in the same fashion as if I were not part of this study. "[66] In other words, this massive study and any complications are to be underwritten by insurance programs in general—that is, if a woman has insurance. And if a woman has no insurance, who will cover the costs? The public?

Breast Cancer Action Group, based in San Francisco, published "Tamoxifen update: Debunking a wonder drug." Adverse effects from tamoxifen include: cancer, increased blood clotting, possible eye damage, liver damage, depression, memory loss, and fatigue.[67] The last may be the hardest to bear for a woman with cancer, already overburdened and stressed.

Given the protocol's stated risks of 62 breast cancers prevented, while causing 38 uterine cancers, and three deaths due to blood clots in the lungs, does the arithmetic make sense? Sixty-two minus 38 uterine cancers, minus 3 blood clot deaths equals a net of 21. According to Michael DeGregorio at the University of Texas Health Science Center in San Antonio, the official study underestimates the chances of fatal blood clot by more than 2 1/2 times, and underestimates that of uterine cancer by 50%.[68]

The estimated risks are stated above. In actuality, the NCI results were 116 breast cancers, including 3 deaths in the tamoxifen group, and 213 breast cancers and 8 deaths in the placebo group. For uterine cancer, there were 33 women in the tamoxifen group versus 14 in controls; for pulmonary embolism there were 17 cases in the tamoxifen group versus 6 in the controls; and for deep vein thrombosis, 30 women in the tamoxifen group versus 19 in the controls. For the last three life-threatening illnesses, the occurrence was 80 in the tamoxifen group versus 39 in the control group. Can this be called disease substitution?

ZENECA, ICI, AND CHEMICALS

Zeneca Corporation was a June 1993 creation of its parent company ICI, one of the world's largest chemical corporations. Zeneca is the marketing agent for tamoxifen, trade named Nolvadex. A mere 0. 39% of shareholders (1108 by number) held 82.1% of Zeneca stock. According to corporate financial reports, these few people owned between 50,001 to more than 1 million shares each. The boards of directors of both ICI and Zeneca are each chaired by Sir Denys Henderson, with nearly 10% of the stock in Zeneca owned by board members.[69] This concentration of decision-making power is made graphic by a 1993 Zeneca Annual Report photograph of the board of directors, which shows 11 figures in nearly identical dark suits, with a lone woman director, also wearing the dark suit "uniform."

From 1992 to 1993, Zeneca, the new subsidiary of ICI, showed a 42% increase in "profit before exceptional items and taxation."[70] Pharmaceutical and agrochemical chemicals accounted for 42% and 33% of its 1993 business. In its "current sales range" of pharmaceuticals for cancer are Nolvadex, its trade name for tamoxifen, and Zoladex (goserelin). The first is prescribed to women with breast cancer, the latter, an inhibitor of pituitary sex hormone release, is prescribed to men with prostate cancer. Eight additional chemicals mentioned under the category of "cancer" are not fully identified, listed as they are by trade name and code numbers.

Zeneca, fourth in world sales of agricultural chemicals, awarded Cambridge University's chemistry department U. S. $1. 9 million over 5 years to discover new compounds, primarily for its pharmaceutical and agrochemical businesses.[71] Zeneca has teamed up with California-based DNA Plant Technology to develop gene technology to produce a "better banana."[72]

On another level, is Zeneca's purchase of Salick Health Care Inc., a chain of 11 cancer treatment centers, worth $438 million. Los Angeles–based Salick Health Care runs the largest for-profit cancer clinic chain in the United States.[73] Zeneca spokesman David Barnes said "The prime motive is that this takes us into disease management as opposed to selling pharmaceutical products."[74]

A month's supply of 60 tamoxifen 10-mg tablets is priced in the United States at $78. 99 and in Yugoslavia $23. 33. From a commercial pharmacy in Canada[75] the same supply can be bought for $17. 81. Those prices are for the generic product. Nolvadex, the Zeneca name-brand product, costs $85.99 for a 1 month's supply in the United States. Now the most widely prescribed cancer medication in the world, it generated in 1992 revenues in the United States of $265 million.[76] Worldwide sales of Nolvadex reached $400 million by 1993, and by 1997, revenues were $508,000,000, about half of which came from sales to women in the United States. Over the April 1998 weekend when the NCI tamoxifen study results were publicized, Zeneca stock rose from $137. 25 to $147. 00.[77]

How smoothly the names Nolvadex and Zoladex roll off the tongue . . . soothing, nonthreatening sounds. . . . And Evista, the next estrogen-blocking drug to be tested, manufactured by Eli Lilly. Contrast the sound of those names with the names from Zeneca's agrochemical division, the herbicides, which account for over 50% of that division's sales: Eradicane, Sutan, Mikado, Fusilade, Grasp, Achieve, Boxer, Touchdown, Devrinol, and Racer. The insecticides include such aggressive names as Force, Dyfonate, Ambush, Karate, and Cymbush. The creative fungicide names include Anvil, Nimrod, Impact, and Captan. As long ago as 1977, Captan was under review by the U.S. EPA when studies showed Captan caused cancer and birth defects and produced both metagenic and chromosomal damage.[78,79] Zeneca's herbicide, Molinate, is under study in humans because of adverse reproductive effects in rodents.[80] Not to be outdone in names is a product in Zeneca's Specialties Division, one called Deepshaft. See Table 9.1.

An implied concern is that Zeneca, a corporate entity, may be manipulating the breast cancer message to divert attention from the issue that some of the chemicals it, and its corporate allies, produce may be contributing to the cancer epidemic. Realistically, with few exceptions, manufacture and promo-

Table 9.1

ZENECA AGRICULTURAL PRODUCTS
(Not all Zeneca/ICI products are included)

	Trade Name	Generic Name	Solubility
Herbicides:			
	Eradicane	Same	Organics
	Sutan	butylate	organics
	Mikado	unknown	
	Fusilade	fluazifop-*p*-ethyl	unknown
	Grasp	tralkoxydim	organics
	Achieve	same as Grasp	
	Boxer	pyrifenox	organics
	Touchdown	glyphosate-trimesium	water
	Racer	unknown	
	Ordram	molinate	organics
Insecticides:			
	Force	tefluthrin	organics
	Ambush	permethrin	organics
	Karate	lambda-cyhalothrin	organics
	Cymbush	cypermethrin	organics
	Demon	cypermethrin	organics
	Lindane	(patented 1940)	organics
Fungicides:			
	Anvil	hexaconazole	organics
	Nimrod	bupirimate	organics
	Impact	flutriafol	organics
	Captan	captan	organics/ low in water
A product of Zeneca's Specialties Division is called			
	Deepshaft	unknown	unknown

Solubility is indicated. Chemicals taken up by organic solvents indicate those that pass readily through the intact skin. Solubility in organic chemicals is also a measure of the ability of the product to partition into and be stored within fat portions of the body.

tion of products, both therapeutic and causative of disease, are an integral part of nearly every major chemical corporation. Zeneca/ICI is no exception.

ICI/Zeneca's underwriting of Breast Cancer Awareness Month (BCAM) is complex. On the board of BCAM are persons from 13 institutions, including the National Cancer Institute, the American Cancer Society, Avon, Estee Lauder, and Hanes.[81] Zeneca contributed $600,000 to endow a professorship at the University of Pittsburgh, in honor of Dr. Bernard Fisher, director of the NSABP trials. In the United States, at least $60 million in tax funds have been awarded for the breast cancer prevention trial. These funds do not include expenditures of insurance costs or "other" medical aspects of the trials that may occur as a result of tamoxifen use.

Early work on tamoxifen was done by Craig Jordan, a pharmacologist currently at Northwestern University in Evanston, Illinois. His research, supported by ICI, showed that tamoxifen did not destroy all of the hormone-dependent tumor cells. Jordan's test animals demonstrated that when tamoxifen "has been cleared from the rat and the normal cyclic hormonal environment returns, the malignant cells are reactivated and develop into palpable tumors."[82] A quote of Jordan in a 1994 issue of *Science*— "Tamoxifen is the only thing we've got now for preventing breast cancer"—has been challenged by others concerned about tamoxifen's ability to damage DNA and cause mutations in the livers of test animals.[83] What must be challenged also is the issue of ignoring primary prevention.

The National Women's Health Network, concerned women, and numerous physicians and scientists have raised significant concerns that must be addressed. The tamoxifen trial is unique: experimental testing upon disease-free women in the face of known adverse effects that have been demonstrated in other women and in test animals. Heretofore, FDA has required that drugs be both efficacious and safe before being administered to humans. And even when a drug risked harm, it was considered appropriate to allow a drug treatment only when the benefit outweighed the risk to the patient. In the context of the tamoxifen trials, this is not treatment.

Nor are the tamoxifen trials primary prevention: chemical castration is not the same as primary prevention. [While castration refers specifically to males, there is no comparable word for females.] Essentially, tamoxifen produces chemical ablation of the ovaries, complete with the signs and symptoms of menopause—not exactly a desirable situation in a woman under the age of normal menopause especially if the antiestrogen effects include acceleration of bone mineral loss and osteoporosis as some have found.[84] To date, no one has suggested a parallel clinical trial on men, achieving hormonal ablation of testicular function to "prevent" prostatic cancer.

Have we progressed? If one has an estrogen-dependent breast cancer, taking a pill twice a day is less physically traumatic than having ones' ovaries surgically removed. But is it? If a woman may develop uterine cancer in addition to breast cancer, can that woman withstand the additional disease, the additional stress?

The tamoxifen trial could very well become a disaster. The potential consequences are life-threatening. The very design, enrolling women at different sites, overseen by many different physicians in different settings, from university centers to private practices, is fraught with record-keeping problems and lack of consistency from group to group. There is no assurance that each and every woman enrolled in the trial is receiving regular and adequate gynecological examinations, eye exams, liver function tests, and blood tests. Ultimately, one must question whether experimentation with a toxic agent that may result in disease substitution rather than disease prevention is ethical.[85] Of equal importance is the lack of uniform followup and record keeping for women taking tamoxifen for treatment of breast cancer.

British scientists, also conducting tamoxifen trials, were critical of the decision to prematurely stop the United States study, citing too few women followed for too short a period of time, and the occurrence of serious side effects.[86] Overall, only 57% of women were kept in the study for 4 or more years. Of these, but 3% were minority women. Some women, enrolled as late as September 1997, received either tamoxifen or a placebo for less than 6 months when the study ended. These factors will make any independent assessment very difficult. Interviewed after the study ended, some women expressed their intention to immediately begin taking tamoxifen. With such an indeterminate end for the study, adverse effects, including breast cancer, developed by the women will be difficult to track and will simply melt into the overall picture of ill health.

The legal aspects of tamoxifen use alone are formidable, citing not only ethics, but a human rights issue. Seattle attorney Leonard Schroeter, whose comments before the House Subcommittee on Human Resources and Intergovernmental Relations hearings were: "[A]ny person who is harmed . . . [by] these trials without first having been fully informed of [tamoxifen's] risks, most probably has an appropriate lawsuit against both the dispensing doctor and the government.[87] "Mr. Schroeter expressed concern that civil rights violations continue to occur because of lack of informed consent, giving examples ranging from the nuclear radiation experiments to current drug tests and medical procedures.[88] He comes by his civil rights concerns justly, having worked with Justice Thurgood Marshall on the school desegregation issue following his graduation from Harvard Law School.

Concern was echoed by then NIH director Bernadine Healey, who stated: "We do not conduct trials without believing, based on scientific evidence, that those [involved] will reap more benefits than undergo risk."[89] In the context of the current antiregulatory climate, one may have a legitimate worry about oversight. Few are aware there is no overall policy at NIH to regulate oversight of clinical trials; some multicenter clinical trials sponsored by NIH do not include on-site data audits; audits of large trials under NCI are required only once every 3 years; and the FDA has no regulation stipulating that a study sponsor conduct regular on-site audits of trial data.[90]

Clinical trials conducted by pharmaceutical corporations carry their own set of problems. These range from using multiple physicians (many with variable knowledge and experience, and some with no training at all in research procedures and overseeing clinical trials); to misinterpretation of data; to the question of outcome and ownership of data; to ignorance; to misrepresentation and fraud.[91] These last two involved submission of fraudulent data to the NSABP by Dr. Roger Poisson from St. Luc Hospital in Montreal.[92,93]

The NCI has recommended that women who take tamoxifen to prevent the recurrence of cancer should not continue the drug for more than 5 years. In October 1998, the Food and Drug Adminstration approved tamoxifen use "to reduce the incidence of breast cancer." Note, Zeneca was not allowed to use the P-word, that is, prevention. What does this mean? Just how long should a woman without breast cancer take this drug? Will a theoretical decrease in breast cancer be offset by an increase in uterine cancer; blood clots leading to fatal pulmonary embolism; liver abnormalities and perhaps cancer; cataract and other eye changes; depression; and premature menopause? Who will know? Who is keeping track? It appears that no one is keeping track, which may be quite acceptable to some, for how will a woman be able to prove that her illness resulted from her use of tamoxifen if no data are collected Although notification to discontinue tamoxifen after 5 years was sent to 22,000 physicians treating cancer patients, there is no indication that other physicians, noncancer specialists, prescribing tamoxifen for treatment or "prevention" were notified. As many as 20% of the 1 million women in the United States prescribed tamoxifen may have been taking the drug more than 5 years.[94]

The tamoxifen trials avoid the bigger issue: prevention of disease in the first place. In classical disease control, taught in schools of medicine and public health, prevention means removal or isolation of an inciting agent.

These methods include such measures as sanitation to prevent contamination of a water supply; mandated pasteurization of milk to kill tuberculosis bacillus; restricted use of liver-damaging carbon tetrachloride as a general solvent; and guard rails to prevent falls from high places. In the case of breast cancer, prevention should take precedence, and that is to control and stop environmental pollution—both chemical and radiological.

I urge the reader not to take my word on these issues, but to do your own research, and maintain a high level of suspicion. When asked if women should take tamoxifen based upon the breast cancer trial results, the answer from NCI is "The decision to take tamoxifen is an individual one in which the benefits and risks of the therapy must be considered."Does this not sound like the Premarin message, placing a medical decision on the women, few of whom have sufficient scientific background to make an informed decision?

Why is our primary, well-funded National Cancer Institute not devoting its efforts to primary prevention? Has breast cancer, like so many aspects of our culture, become just another business opportunity?

From the time of Hippocrates, the aim of medicine has been to place caution first and "do no harm." Such costly ventures as promoting drugs to block hormones in healthy women diverts attention, scarce resources, and funding away from **preventing** cancer in the first place.

REFERENCES

1. Evidence of the Carcinogenicity of Tamoxifen. Reproductive and Cancer Assessment Section. Office of Environmental Health Assessment. California Environmental Protection Agency. 39 pages. March 1995.
2. State of California, Environmental Protection Agency, Office of Environmental Health Hazard Assessment, Safe Drinking Water and Toxic Enforcement Act of 1996: Chemicals Known to the State to Cause Cancer or Reproductive Toxicity. Listed September 1, 1996, page 6 of the Revised list of May 1, 1997.
3. Public Forum on Tamoxifen Comments 12/4/1995, Office of Environmental Health Hazard Assessment, Science Advisory Board, 601 North 7th Street, Sacramento, CA 94234-7370.
4. Press Release, National Institutes of Health, April 6, 1998. The letterhead logo says: "Cancer Research—Because lives depend on it."
5. Breast Cancer Trials Committee,Adjuvant tamoxifen in the management of operable breast cancer. Lancet. 2: 171–175, 1987.
6. Fisher, B., and 20 other authors. Five versus more than five years of tamoxifen therapy for breast cancer patients with negative lymph nodes and estrogen

receptor-positive tumors. J. Nat. Cancer Inst. 99(21): 1529–1542, 1996.

7. Jonat, W., Maass, H. The present status of the adjuvant endocrine treatment. J. Steroid Biochem. 27: 499–502, 1987.

8. Nomura, Y., Miura, S., Koyama, H., Enomoto, K., Kasumi, F., Yamamoto, H., Kimura, M., Tominaga, I., Iiona, H., Morimoto, T., Tashiro, H. Relative effect of steroid hormone receptors on the prognosis of patients with operable breast cancer. Cancer. 69: 153–164, 1991.

9. Lear, L. Rachel Carson—Witness for Nature, Henry Holt and Co.. New York. pp. 478–479. 1997.

10. Fisher. Op. cit.

11. Jaiyesimi, I. A., Buzdar, A.U., Decker, D. A., Hortobagyi, G.N. Use of tamoxifen for breast cancer: Twenty-eight years later. J. Clin. Oncol. 13(2): 513–529, 1995.

12. "Dear Doctor" letter from Zeneca Pharmaceuticals Group. 3 pages. April 8, 1994.

13. van Leeuwen, F. E., Benraadt, J., Coebergh, J. W. W., Kiemeney, L. A. L. M., Gimbrere, C. H. F., Otter, R., Schouten, L. J., Damhuis, R. A. M., Bontenbal, M., Diepenhorst, F. W., van den Belt-Dusebout, A. W., van Tinteren, H. Risk of endometrial cancer after tamoxifen treatment of breast cancer. Lancet. 343: 448–452, 1994.

14. Kedar, R.P., Bourne, T. H., Powles, T. J., Collins, W. P., Ashley, S. E., Cosgrove, D. O., Campbell, S. Effects of tamoxifen on uterus and ovaries of postmenopausal women in a randomized breast cancer prevention trial. Lancet. 343: 1318–1321, 1994.

15. Marshall, E. Tamoxifen: Hanging in the balance. Science. 264: 1524–1527, 1994.

16. Nease, R. F., Ross, J. M. The decision to enter a randomized trial of tamoxifen for the prevention of breast cancer in health women: An analysis of the tradeoffs. Amer. J. Med. 99: 180–189, 1995.

17. Cohen, J. Clinical trial monitoring: Hit or miss? Science. 264: 1534–1537, 1994.

18. Op. cit. NCI April 5, 1998.

19. Furr, B. J. A., Jordan, V. C. The pharmacology and clinical uses of tamoxifen. Pharmacol. Therapeut. 25: 127–205, 1984.

20. Bulger, W. H., Muccitelli, R. M., Kupfer, D. Studies on the induction of rat uterine ornithine decarboxylase by DDT analogs. II. Kinetic characteristics of ornithene carboxylase induced by DDT analogs and estradiol. Pestic. Biochem. Physiol. 8(3): 263–270, 1978.

21. Wassermann, M., Nogueira, D. P., Tomatis, L., Mirra, A.P., Shibata, H., Arie, G., Cucos, S., Wassermann, D. Organochlorine compounds in neoplastic and adjacent apparently normal breast tissue. Bull. Environ. Contam. Toxicol. 15(4): 478–484, 1976.

22. Bitman, J., Cecil, H. C., Harris, S. J., Fries, G. F. Estrogenic activity of o,p´-DDT in the mammalian uterus and avian oviduct. Science. 162: 371–372, 1968.

23. Heinrichs, W. L., Geller, R. J., Bakke, J. L. Lawrence, N. L. DDT administered to neonatal rats induces persistent estrus syndrome. Science. 173(997): 642–643, 1971.

24. Shabad, L. M., Kolesnichenko, T. A., Nikonova, T. V. Transplacental and combined long-term effect of DDT in five generations of A-strain mice. Internat. J. Cancer. 11(3): 688–693, 1973.

25. Turusov, V. S., Day, N. E., Tomatis, L., Gati, E., Charles, R. T. Tumors in CF—a mice exposed for six generations to DDT. J. Nat. Cancer Inst. 51(3): 983–997, 1973.

26. Wolff, M. Blood levels of organochlorine residues and risk of breast cancer. N. Nat. Cancer Inst. 85: 648–652, 1993.

27. Sherman, J. D. Chemical Exposure and Disease. Princeton Scientific Publishing Co., Inc. Princeton, NJ. pp. 33, 46, 68,122–123, 173–188. 1994.

28. Shimkin, M. B., Grady, H. G. Carcinogenic potency of stilbestrol and estrone in strain C3H mice. J. Nat. Cancer Inst. 1: 119–128, 1941.

29. Herbst, A. L., Scully, R. E. Adenocarcinoma of the vagina in adolescence. Cancer. 25: 745–757, 1970.

30. Vorheer, H., Messer, R. H., Vorheer, U. F., Jordan, S. W., Kornfeld, M. Teratogenesis and carcinogenesis in rat offspring after transplacental and transmammary exposure to diethylstilbestrol. Biochem. Pharmacol. 28(12): 1864–1877, 1979.

31. Cunha, G. R., Taguchi, O., Namikawa, R. Teratogenic effects of clomiphene, tamoxifen, and diethylstilbestrol on the developing female tract. Human Pathol. 18: 1132–1143, 1987.

32. Zeneca "Dear Doctor" letter of 2 April, 1994. Hardell, L. Tamoxifen as a risk factor for carcinoma of the corpus uteri. Lancet. 2: 563, 1988.

33. Nicholson, R. I., Griffiths, K. The biochemistry of tamoxifen action. Adv. Sex Hormone Res. 4: 119–152, 1980.

34. Jordan, V. C., Dix, C. J., Naylor, K. E. Nonsteroidal antiestrogens: Their biological effects and potential mechanisms of action. J. Toxicol. Environ. Health. 4(2–3): 363–390, 1978.

35. Fornander, T., Rutqvist, L. E., Cedarmark, B., Glas, U. Adjuvant tamoxifen in early breast cancer: occurrence of new primary cancers. Lancet. 1: 117–120, 1989.

36. Cohen, I., Altara, M. M., Tepper, R., Cordoba, M., Figer, A., Zalel, Y., Dror, Y., Beyth, Y. Different coexisting endometrial histological features in asymptomatic postmenopausal breast cancer patient treated with tamoxifen. Gynecol. Obstet. Investig. 43: 60–63, 1997.

37. Exacoustos, C., Zupi, E., Cangi, B., Chiaretti, M., Ardini, D., Romanini, C. Endometrial evaluation in postmenopausal breast cancer patients receiving tamoxifen: an ultrasound, color flow Doppler, hysteroscopic and histological study. Ultrasound Obstet. Gynecol. 6: 435–442, 1995.

38. Tate, A. C., Lieberman, M. E., Jordan, V. C. The inhibition of prolactin synthesis in GH3 rat pituitary tumor cells by monohydroxytamoxifen in associated with changes in the properties of the estrogen receptor. J. Steroid Biochem. 20: 391–395, 1984.

39. Danielian, P. S., White, R., Hoare, S. A., Fawell, S. E., Parker, M. G.

Identification of residues in the estrogen receptor that confer differential sensitivity to estrogen and hydroxytamoxifen. Molec. Endocrinol. 7: 232–240, 1993.

40. Jordan, V. C., Murphy, C. S. Endocrine pharmacology of antiestrogens as antitumor agents. Endocrine Rev. 11: 578–610, 1990.

41. Kedar, R. P., Bourne, T. H., Powles, T. J. Effects of tamoxifen on uterus and ovaries of postmenopausal women in a randomized breast cancer prevention trial. Lancet. 343: 1318–1321, 1994.

42. Fisher, B., Constantino, J. P., Redmond, C. K., et al. Endometrial cancer in tamoxifen-treated breast cancer patients: findings from the National Surgical Adjuvant Breast and Bowel Project (NASBP) B-14. J. Nat. Cancer Inst. 86: 527–537, 1994.

43. Philips, D. H., Venitt, S. Safety of prophylactic tamoxifen. Lancet. 341: 1485–1486, 1993.

44. Mani, C., Kupfer, D. Cytochrome P-450 mediated action and irreversible binding of the antiestrogen tamoxifen to proteins in rat and human liver: possible involvment of the flavin-containing monooxygenases in tamoxifen activaiton. Cancer Res. 51: 6052–6058, 1991.

45. Harper, M. J. K., Walpole, A. L. Contrasting endocrine activities of cis and trans isomers in a series of substituted triphenylethylenes. Nature. 21: 87, 1966.

46. Harper, M. J. K., Walpole, A. L. Mode of action of ICI 46,474 in preventingimplantation in rats. J. Endocrinol. 37: 83–92, 1967.

47. U. S. Food and Drug Administration. Bulletin. p. 3. May 1994.

48. Kristensen, B., Ejlertsen, B., Mouridsen, H. T., Andersen, K. W., Lauritzen, J. B. Femoral fractures in postmenopausal breast cancer patients treated with adjuvant tamoxifen. Breast Cancer Res. Treatment. 39: 321–326, 1996.

49. NCI. April 6, 1998.

50. Tewari, K., Bonebrake, R. G., Asrat, T., Shanberg, A. M. Ambiguous genitalia in infant exposed to tamoxifen in utero. Lancet. 350: 183, 1997.

51. Luster, M. I., Faith, R. E., McLachlan, J. A., Clark, G. C. Effect of in utero exposure to diethylstilbestrol on the immune response in mice. Toxicol. Appl. Pharmacol. 47(2): 279–285, 1979.

52. Nicholson, R. I., Griffiths, K. The biochemistry of tamoxifen action. Adv. Sex Hormone Res. 4: 119–152, 1980.

53. Fendl, K. C., Zimniski, S. J. Role of tamoxifen in induction of hormone-independent rat mammary tumors. Cancer Res. 52: 235–237, 1992.

54. Physicians' Desk Reference. Medical Economics Co. Inc. Montvale, NJ. pp. 1126–1128. 1993.

55. Fentiman, I. S. Tamoxifen and mastalgia. Drugs. 32: 477–480, 1986.

56. Information about this and other advocacy groups is listed in Chapter 17.

57. Pavlidia, N. A., Petris, C., Briassoulis, E. Clear evidence that long-term low-dose tamoxifen treatment can induce ocular toxicity. Cancer. 69: 2961–2964, 1992.

58. Bentley, C. R., Davies, G., Aclimondos, W. A. Tamoxifen retinopathy, a rare but serious complication. Brit. Med. J. 304: 495–496, 1992.

59. Vinding, T., Nielsen, N. V. Retinopathy caused by treatment with tamoxifen in low dose. Acta Opthalmol. 61: 45–50, 1983.

60. Zhang, J. J., Jacob, Y. J., Valverde, M. A., Hardy, S. P., Minteng, G. M., Sepulveda, F. V., Gill, D. R., Hyde, S. C., Trezise, A. E., Higgins, C. F. Tamoxifen blocks chloride channels. A possible mechanism for cataract formaiton. J. Clin. Investig. 94(4): 1690–1697, 1994.

61. Fugh-Berman, A., Pearson, C., Rennie, S. Food and Drug Administration Oncological Drugs Advisory Committee: Proposed Tamoxifen Prevention Trial. 9 pages. July 2, 1991.

62. National Women's Health Network. NWHN responds to NCI announcement of "Good News. " What about prevention for the rest of us? 514 10th Street, N. W., Suite 400, Washington, D. C. 20004. 2 pages. April 6, 1998.

63. Pavlidis, N. A., Petris, C., Briasoulis, E. Clear evidence that long-term, low-dose tamoxifen treatment can induce ocular toxicity. Cancer. 69: 2961–2964, 1992.

64. Fisher, B., Constantino, J. P., Redmond, C. K., Fisher, E. R., Wickerham, D. L., Cronin, W. M. Endometrial cancer in tamoxifen-treated breast cancer patients: Findings from the National surgical adjuvant breast and bowel projects (NSABP) B-14. J. Nat. Cancer Inst. 86: 527–537, 1994.

65. Bissett, D., Davis, J. A., George, W. D. Gynecological monitoring during tamoxifen therapy. Lancet. 344: 1244, 1994.

66. Fisher, B., University of Pittsburgh. Consent to act as a participant in a clinical trial. 7 pages January 1, 1992.

67. Evans, N. Tamoxifen Update: Debunking a wonder drug. Breast Cancer Action, Newsletter #35. p. 1. April 1996.

68. DeGregorio, M. W. Is tamoxifen chemoprevention worth the risk in healthy women? J. NIH Research. 4: 84–87, 1992.

69. Zeneca Annual Report and Accountants. 68 pages. 1993.

70. US FDA. Op. cit.

71. Pesticide Action Network. Global Pesticide Campaigner. 5(3): 19, 1995. Available from PAN, 116 New Montgomery, Suite 810, San Francisco, CA 94105.

72. Cole, R. Banana is latest food with biotech upgrade. Kalamazoo Gazette. p. A-8. July 9, 1994.

73. Firshein, J. Drug firm buys up chain of US cancer clinics. Lancet. 349: 1230, 1997.

74. Hilzenrath, D. S. Drugmaker to enter care field. Washington Post. p. B-2. December 23, 1994.

75. WalMart Pharmacy, Kingston, Ontario.

76. Rock, A. The breast cancer experiment. Ladies Home Journal. pp. 144–151. February, 1995.

77. Okie, S. Tamoxifen lowers risk of breast cancer. Washington Post Health page 7 April 7, 1998.

78. US EPA, RPAR (Rebutable Presumption Against Registration) for Captan. August 10, 1977.

79. US EPA, Substitute Chemical Program, Initial Scientific and Minieconomic

Review of Captan, EPA-540/1-75-012. 173 pages. April, 1975.

80. Bureau National Affairs 92: A-4, May 14, 1996.

81. It was Lauder's division, Origins, that supplied the chemically laden cosmetic "gift" at a Breast Cancer Awareness luncheon.

82. Jordan, V. C., Allen, K. E., Dix, C. J. Pharmacology of tamoxifen in laboratory animals. Cancer Treatment Reports. 64(6–7): 745–759, 1980.

83. Seachrist, L. Animal tests take back seat to clinical data. Science. 264: 1525, 1994.

84. Gotfredson, A., Christiansen, C., Palshof, T. The effect of tamoxifen on bone mineral content in premenopausal women with breast cancer. Cancer. 53: 853–857, 1984.

85. Fugh-Berman, A., Epstein, S. Tamoxifen: disease prevention or disease substitution. Lancet. 340: 1143–1147, 1992.

86. Reaney, P. UK doctors criticize US handling of cancer study. Reuters, London. April 7, 1998.

87. Raloff, J. Tamoxifen and informed consent/dissent. Sci. News. 142: 378–340, 1992.

88. Schroeter, L. W. Personal communication. April 10, 1998.

89. Raloff. Op. cit.

90. Cohen, J. Clinical trial monitoring: Hit or miss? Science 264: 1534–1537, 1994.

91. Nowak, R. Problems in clinical trials go far beyond misconduct. Science. 264: 1538–1541, 1994.

92. Cohen. Op. cit.

93. Fisher, B., Constantino, J. P., Redmond, C. K., Fisher, E. R., Wickerham, D. L., Cronin, W. M., and other NSABP Contributors. [12 additional contributors from the U. S. and Canada are listed at end of article]. Endometrial cancer in tamoxifen-treated breast cancer patients: Findings from the National Surgical Adjuvant Breast and Bowel Project (NSABP) B-14. J. Nat. Cancer Inst. 86(7): 527–537, 1994.

94. Brown, D. Study backs 5-year limit on breast cancer drug. Washington Post. p. A-28. December 1, 1995.

10

POST-MENOPAUSAL HORMONE REPLACEMENT
QUESTIONS AND RISKS

YOUNG FOREVER

The view of menopause as an abnormality to be corrected is not new. In 1937, the respected *British Medical Journal* carried a popular and revealing article:

> Practically every menopausal woman becomes aware of a certain mental clumsiness, and inability to cope with the ordinary problems of daily life, and a tendency to "give in." *The realization of her shortcomings* is worrying and she readily becomes depressed. Emotional instability is well defined, and the patient reacts to trivial situations with rather surprising attacks of laughter or tears. She is subject to rapid and frequent changes of mood: at one moment she will be unbearably irritable, at the next pathetically contrite. There may be marked changes in personality and severe attacks of mental depression, sometimes lasting for days, during which the patient becomes suicidal. A condition of hypochondriasis, which is *particularly distressing to those around her*, may develop out of the complicated syndrome, even in the milder cases, and persist for the remainder of the patient's life.[1] (Emphasis added.)

The recommended "treatment" was, of course, estrogen therapy, and as recently as 1987, DES was still being promoted for post-menopausal symptoms.[2]

Continuing today, if you are approaching menopause, you may be given a full-color video tape by Wyeth-Ayerst Corporation and an artistically designed packet containing sample tablets of Premarin. Wyeth-Ayerst bills itself as providing "Worldwide Leadership in Female Healthcare," which has a ring of truth, since more than 5 million women currently take Premarin, a chemical doctors prescribe 6 times more frequently than any other estrogen product.[3]

The "conjugated estrogens" material, trademarked as Premarin, was first patented in 1951. Premarin contains an amorphous mix of hormones, obtained from the urine of pregnant mares. Similar products carry names such as Amnestrogen, Conestron, Estrifol, and Genisis. Despite the non-threatening sound of the names, since at least 1985 these products have been classified as carcinogens.[4]

In bold print, the Wyeth-Ayerst booklet on Premarin states: "Majority of studies have not shown an increased risk of breast cancer with low doses of estrogen used after menopause." However, one needs to read the fine print. And fine print it is: a 2 1/2 inch by 31 inch package insert, which for a menopausal woman (a person over the age of 50) may be difficult to impossible to read. In part, it states:

> Some studies have suggested a possible increased incidence of breast cancer in those women on estrogen therapy taking higher doses for prolonged periods of time. The majority of studies, however, have not shown an association with the usual doses used for estrogen replacement therapy. . . . The reported endometrial cancer risk among estrogen users was about 4-fold or greater than in nonusers and appears dependent on duration of treatment and on estrogen dose. There is not significant increased risk associated with the use of estrogens for less than one year. The greatest risk appears associated with prolonged use—five years or more. In one study, persistence of risk was demonstrated for 10 years after cessation of estrogen treatment.[5]

The wording in the most recent company release reads essentially the same as above. Added in bold print is the caution: "Estrogens have been reported to increase the risk of endometrial carcinoma in postmenopausal women."[6]

The adverse effects from post-menopausal use of estrogens have been well documented. There is an increased risk in uterine (endometrial) cancer after only 2 years of use, and a 20-fold increase after 10 to 15 years of estrogen replacement therapy. The elevated risk remained whether the regimen was cyclic or not, and whether conjugated or other forms of estrogens were prescribed.[7] There is a problem in determining the true incidence of uterine cancer. Many women undergo hysterectomies (removal of the uterus) for conditions unrelated to uterine cancer, thus altering the statistics.

In an attempt to make sense of the many studies that have been conducted on the risk of breast cancer and post-menopausal hormone use, researchers conducted an analysis of data from 51 epidemiological studies from 21 countries, mostly in North America and Europe. Included for analysis were 52,705 women with breast cancer and 108,411 women without a diagnosis of breast cancer. The longer the duration of use of hormonal therapy, the larger the cumulative excess numbers of breast cancers. In this study group, women between the ages of 50 and 70 who had never used post-menopausal hormones had an incidence ranging from 18 to 63 per 1000 women. The taking of post-menopausal hormones for 5 years, increases the cumulative excess by 2 per 1000 women; for 10 years the increase is 6 cases per 1000; and for 15 years the excess number of cases is 12 for every 1000 users. The authors calculate that post-menopausal hormone use for 4 years would result in one extra breast cancer being diagnosed in every 1000 users, and use for 13 years would result in one additional breast cancer in every 100 users.[8]

Which among the many components of Premarin are cancer-causing is not known for sure, but when one component (equilenin) was mixed with DNA, the result was the formation of abnormal metabolites.[9] Complicating the diagnosis of breast cancer in a woman taking post-menopausal hormones is the suggestion that hormone therapy delays diagnosis by increasing the density of the breast, thus making lesions more difficult to detect by mammography.[10]

Further complication the issue of Premarin usage is that it is supplied in tablets ranging in dose from 0.3 to 2.4 mg. The latter dose contains 8 times more of the drug than the lowest dose, and women are frequently prescribed varying dosages throughout a period of treatment. The package insert, supplied directly to women, leaves vague the recommended dose of estrogen and duration of use. Rather, it says: "You must decide, with your doctor, whether the risk of estrogens are acceptable in view of their benefits."

This is a curious twist of language. In medical matters, one usually considers risk in terms of benefits, not harm. The package insert continues: "The length of treatment with estrogens will depend upon the reason for use. This should also be discussed with your doctor." This tactic places an inordinate burden upon a woman to act as her own pharmacologist. It makes it no less simple for the physician, or for a woman knowledgeable in pharmacology and toxicology, for no bibliographic sources are given. It's impossible to verifythe message.

Despite these well-established adverse findings, lack of information concerning alternative health measures, and the entire question of whether it is appropriate for post-menopausal women to take hormones at all, there is still a push to promote these products, even for women with breast cancer.

Dr. Melody Cobleigh and associates of Rush-Presbyterian-St. Luke's Medical Center in Chicago wrote "We believe that the time is right to study the effects of estrogen replacement therapy" in breast cancer survivors.[11] This may bring an unwanted outcome for women with cancer: what *if* hormonal use results in acceleration of cancer? Will the "potential" benefit of estrogen replacement hasten the deaths of women already suffering with breast cancer? Who will benefit from this type of experiment, the woman or a seller of drugs? Who will suffer? And who will answer for the consequences? These questions are yet unanswered, but they ought to be.

Women are bombarded by articles in the popular press that tout the use of hormone replacement therapy but don't resolve the issues. The cover of the June 1995 Time magazine announced "Estrogen—Every Woman's Dilemma" and portrayed the photograph of a hand belonging to a young woman on the left, and the hand of an older person on the right. What we aren't told is how much work the hand on the right had done, and whether a wrinkle-free life is achievable by taking a pill.

Press releases in July and August 1996 proposed estrogen use to lower the risk of Alzheimer's disease.[12,13] This of course was a little more than a year after another press release that linked estrogen use to breast cancer.[14] Cynically, one wonders if this is a new way to keep the prescriptions flowing. While the media keep estrogens in the spotlight, the scientific debate continues, proposing yet more study.[15] The net effect is that it is difficult for both physicians and women to make an *informed* decision. I emphasize informed, because media hype is no substitute for data derived from independent studies.

Before women accept the concept of post-menopause "therapy,"a number of ideas need consideration. Do most post-menopausal women *need* estrogens at all? Can post-menopausal heart disease and bone loss be controlled with proper diet, calcium supplements, a cessation of smoking, and increasing one's exercise? These measures, as opposed to taking a chemical hormone, have not been adequately studied.

The sellers of these products emphasize the role of estrogens as protection against osteoporosis and heart disease, which undeniably are significant problems. But it is wise to remember that the estrogen industry is in the business of selling products. Is being urged to take a pharmaceutical product for a normal body event motivated by financial gain to the exclusion of safe medical practice?

CONFOUNDING FACTORS

Two reports in the New England Journal of Medicine add to the hormone story.[16,17] These suggest that two alcoholic drinks a day may be enough to raise hormone levels in women, putting them at greater risk for developing breast cancer. Some reports say that women who drink moderately have a breast cancer risk 40 to 100% more than women who don't drink, but no study, correcting for diet, medication intake, exposure to ionizing radiation, and other chemical exposures has been done to ascertain what part alcohol actually contributes to the increase.

We don't know if the alcohol factor is real or another of the "blame-the-victim" arguments, deflecting emphasis away from the sea of hormones and carcinogens in which women are immersed. Either way, it is well to remember that anything that alters normal liver function, such as alcohol use, gall bladder disease, or foreign chemicals that depend upon the liver for metabolism and excretion will slow the removal of chemicals such as DES from the body.[18]

WHAT THEN TO DO, OR NOT DO?

Menopause is a time in a woman's life when it is natural for her hormonal levels to decrease. Thus, it is reasonable to ask if this is a "condition" to be treated at all. A reliable source of information on whether to take hormones after menopausal is a well-documented, peer-reviewed, easy-to-understand booklet prepared by the National Women's Health Network, and the booklet is a realistic antidote to the pharmaceutical industry message. It tells us what hormone replacement cannot do. It cannot prevent signs of aging, wrinkles, heart disease, and Alzheimer's. It cannot improve memory or solve psychological problems. It outlines valid reasons why not to use hormonal products, what common side effects to expect, and finally, outlines what measures ought to be taken before and during any hormonal use.[19]

ESTROGENS AND BREAST CANCER

In summary, factors linking estrogens and cancer are:

1. The higher the daily dose of estrogen, the less time it takes for the development of cancer.
2. A more constant absorption of estrogen reduces both the time for development of cancer as well as the amount of hormone required.
3. The greater the estrogenic potency, the less time required for the development of breast cancer.
4. Estrogenic chemicals of radically different chemical structures similar in their hormonal action are similar in their cancer-producing action.
5. Estrogen administration is associated with a variety of breast cancer cell-types: comedo, ductal, fibroadenomatous, all having the ability to metastasize.
6. Long-term, repeated administration of relatively small doses may intensify tissue responses to a hormonal substance.

The conclusions are quite clear: women (and men) have been the experimental objects of some flawed practices. Corporate and governmental bodies have sanctioned the use of chemicals that have affected our bodies directly and indirectly. The promotional literature urges we women to confer with our doctors to decide if hormone replacement is for us. Does that mean that if we have an adverse outcome as a result of our decision (to use hormone replacement or not to use hormone replacement chemicals) that we will be again blamed for the outcome?

> There are maladies we must not seek to cure because they alone protect us from others that are more serious.
>
> —Proust, *Remembrance of Things Past*

REFERENCES

1. Bishop, P. M. F. Endocrines in theory and practice: The menopause. Brit. Med. J. 819–821, 1937.
2. Physicians' Desk Reference. Medical Economics Co., Inc., Oradell, NJ. p.1136. 1987.
3. Anon. What every woman should know about estrogen. Wyeth-Ayerst Laboratories. Philadelphia. 19 pages. 1991.
4. National Technical Program, Fourth Annual Report on Carcinogens, 85-002. p. 61. 1985.

5. Anon. Package insert for Premarin. Ayerst Laboratories, Inc. New York, NY. Revised March 9, 1990.

6. Physicians' Desk Reference. Medical Economics Co., Inc., Montvale, NJ. p. 3111. 1998.

7. Weiss, N. S., Szekely, D. R., English, D. R., Schweid, A. I. Endometrial cancer in relation to patterns of menopausal estrogen use. J. Amer. Med. Assoc. 242(3): 261–264, 1979.

8. Collaborative Group on Hormone Factors in Breast Cancer. Breast cancer and hormone replacement therapy: collaborative reanalysis of data from 51 epidemiological studies of 52,705 women with breast cancer and 108,411 women without breast cancer. Lancet. 350: 1047–1059, 1997.

9. Wunsch, H. Oestrogen metabolite linked to cancer risk in some hormone replacements. Lancet. 351: 345, 1998.

10. Beral, V., Banks, E., Reeves, G., Wallis, M. Hormone replacement therapy and high incidence of breast cancer between mammographic screens. Lancet. 349:1103–1104, 1997.

11. Anon. Misunderstanding estrogen. Washington Post. p. A-2. August 17, 1994.

12. Brody, J. E, Estrogen therapy studies as Alzheimer's treatment. The Denver Post. p. 3-A. July 21, 1996.

13. Friend, T. Estrogen may lower woman's risk of Alzheimer's. USA Today. p. A-1. August 16–18, 1996.

14. Brown, D. Breast cancer, estrogen link is affirmed. Washington Post. p. A-25. June, 15, 1995.

15. Neven, P., De Muylder, X, Hormonal interventions and cancer risk. Lancet. 346: 8–9. 1995.

16. Schatzkin, A., Jones, D. Y., Hoover, R. N., Taylor, P. R., Brinton, L. A. Ziegler, R. G., Harvey, E. B., Carter, C. L., Licitra, L. M., Dufour, M. C. Alcohol consumption and breast cancer in the epidemiologic follow-up study of the first National Health and Nutritional Examination Survey. New Engl. J. Med. 316(19): 1169–1173, 1987.

17. Willett, W. C., Stampfer, M. J., Colditz, G. A., Rosner, B. A., Hennekens, C. H., Speizer, F. E. Moderate alcohol consumption and the risk of breast cancer. New Engl. J. Med., 316(19): 1174–1180, 1987.

18. Klaassen, C. D. The effect of altered hepatic function on the toxicity, plasma disappearance and biliary excretion of diethylstilbestrol. Toxicol. Appl. Pharmacol. 24: 142–149, 1973.

19. Taking Hormones and Women's Health: Choices, Risks and Benefits. National Women's Health Network, 514 Tenth Street, N.W., Suite 400, Washington, D.C. 20004. 49 pages. 1995.

11

THE GENETIC CONNECTION
BIOLOGY AND
ECONOMIC AND SOCIAL RAMIFICATIONS

We are so curiously made that one atom put in the wrong place in our
original structure will often make us unhappy for life
—William Godwin (1756–1836)

I had initially thought this chapter should be called, Aladdin's genie. Genie
brings to mind a guardian deity, but unfortunately genie has an alternative
meaning, and that is demon.[1] The genie of discovery, the manipulator and
controller of genetic information (same word derivation) we find has been
liberated! Humans and the environment are in peril, and this is no Aladdin
fantasy. Dolly, the cloned sheep, was hyped by the media, and some have
plans to clone humans. The ramifications of genetic science, known, and
more ominously, unknown, bear careful scrutiny.

What can women expect from genetic research—the topic talked about
on every media outlet? An article in the *Journal of the American Medical
Association* discusses gene tests and cancer, diagnosis, measurement of
tumor progression, therapy, and drugs. *At no place in this article on the
"cancer revolution" is primary prevention mentioned.*[2] What can we expect?
Little, unless we demand specific action.

This exploding field of gene manipulation was proclaimed on the cover of
the final 1993 issue of Science, the journal of the American Association for
the Advancement of *Science*. It named "p53, the Molecule of the Year,"
touting it the "genetic key to cancer." Tribute to this life-sustaining factor
was repeated in the same journal a year later, announcing "DNA Repair—
Molecule of the Year."[3]

Sorely misunderstood by being linked to cancer, p53 is not the cause of cancer. No, p53 is a normal and necessary component of life. Its function is to *suppress tumor formation.* p53 must be intact and functional, not injured, to be able to perform its intended protective function, and if it is damaged, it will not work as it is intended.

If the primary aim of genetic research is to prevent cancer, it is essential to link gene abnormalities to cancer-causing agents. Without identification of various carcinogenic stimuli capable of setting in motion the dysfunction of the p53 gene, it is unlikely that the "magic bullet" of gene identification for cancer will be more than an expensive laboratory technique.

Nearly 100% of genetic mutations are called "mis-sense"—damage that results in alteration of a gene that codes for a single amino acid. In other words, the message no longer makes sense, and the resultant "non-sense" must not be regarded as "harm-less."

About half of all cancers, including breast cancers, show mutations in the p53 gene. But mutations of the p53 gene differ with different cancer sites, and mutations are not constant even for cancers of a single organ.[4] For example, people in China with liver cancer showed an entirely different p53 gene pattern from those with the same cancer in the United States. This is undoubtedly due to differences in carcinogenic stimuli in these two very different countries. It is postulated in the case of liver cancer in China that the stimulus is a fungus, common in China, but rare in the United States.[5]

Most mutations of the p53 gene occur in the fatty, called lipophilic, portion of the gene in a small area that binds to DNA.[6] Because many carcinogens thought to be involved in breast and reproductive cancers are lipid-soluble, this mutational pattern strengthens the research link between exposure to such chemicals and cancer. One group of industrial chemicals, all fat-soluble, includes the hormone diethylstilbestrol (DES); many organochlorine pesticides such as chlordane, heptachlor, lindane, aldrin, dieldrin, kepone, DDT; the PCBs; dioxins and dibenzofurans. None of these chemicals is found naturally in nature; all are man-made.

If we are to stop the chemical-cancer link, the type and frequency of gene mutations and body burden of carcinogenic chemicals must be documented. This carcinogen-specific research deserves at least as much effort and financial support as personal gene identification. Given the potential for profit from patented gene-testing, and the threat to the status quo if the chemical pollution–cancer link becomes documented, it is unlikely that the needed research will be undertaken unless there is concerted pressure to do so.

How do cancer mutations come about? Through interference and damage by chemicals and/or various forms of radiation. Some mutations are random and a part of the normal evolutionary process that allows new genetic traits to emerge. The amazing creatures of the Galapagos are examples of what happens when genetic changes occur on an isolated island.

Much of the cancer epidemic of today is a result of increasing exposure to chemical and radiation factors. Although many of us have genetic susceptibility to one illness or another, a second triggering factor from the environment is needed to make the abnormality or disease manifest. Allergies come to mind: the susceptible individual can be symptom-free in the absence of the offending agent, be it ragweed, penicillin, or a cat. Unfortunately, throughout our common evolutionary history, we have not developed mechanisms to respond to many novel, man-made, insults.

Genetic damage is common, judging by the fact that 90% of p53 damages are "mis-sense" mutations, whereby the identity of a single amino acid is changed. Mis-sense changes in p53 are two-edged: resulting in both loss of tumor-*suppressor* activity and a gain of *carcinogenic* function.[7] It is the tumor-suppressor activity that is protective.

Since these mutations occur only after the time of conception and birth, if we were able to test an individual on a daily basis, there would be a day when that person's genetic makeup would be transformed from normal to abnormal. What would be the event or events to cause that remarkable change? At which point in time, on which gene, on which chromosome, and on how many other genes would a change be found? The enormity of identifying that single genetic change from normal to abnormal would make easy finding a needle in a haystack.

What sets those "random" events into motion? Oncogenes operate in all animals, human and nonhuman. All chemicals known to cause cancer in humans cause cancer in animals, without exception. We can look at the following sentence and see how a simple alteration changes meaning, and thus the message:

SHE BROUGHT COURAGE TO SKILL AND HER REASONS.
SHE BROUGHT   RAGE TO SKILL AND HER REASONS.
SHE BROUGHT   RAGE TO KILL AND HER REASONS.
SHE BROUGHT   RAGE TO KILL   HER REASONS.
SHE BROUGHT   RAGE TO KILL   HER   SON.

In just four steps we have transformed a positive and benign statement into a deadly, malignant one. An alteration in a letter, word, sentence, paragraph, or page of text results in garbled, misleading, false, or harmful information. In the same manner, a mutation that is an alteration in a few genes changes the very function and meaning of life.

The article "A strong candidate for the breast and ovarian cancer susceptibility gene BRCA1" received major media attention. It lists the name of 45 authors, and carries an important sentence: "It will be of utmost importance in future studies to identify other genetic factors or environmental factors that may ameliorate the effects of BRCA1 mutations."[8] A companion piece in the same journal concluded: "These results suggest that mutation of BRCA1 may not be critical in the development of the majority of breast cancers that arises in the absence of a mutant germline allele."[9] Unfortunately, since those papers were released, the press has carried precious little information about other genetic or environmental factors that surely are a part of the breast cancer epidemic. Rather, the press and the scientific community have emphasized genetic testing and genetic manipulation.

Work done largely at the University of Utah identified the location of the now famous BRCA1 gene that is associated with an inherited form of breast cancer. It was claimed that BRCA1 (BReast CAncer-1) is the gene responsible for about 5% of the total breast cancer cases. This leaves unaccounted for the 95% of women who develop breast cancer in the absence of this genetic alteration. With the passage of time since the announcement of the breast cancer gene by the Utah researchers, a number of groups of women have been tested. Prevalence of the BRCA1 gene ranged from zero% in black women and 3.3% in white women (each group ages 20 to 74) at time of diagnosis, to 33.3% in a high-risk family, defined as the patient having four or more family members with breast or ovarian cancer. The researchers conclude that for the general United States population, widespread screening was not warranted.[10] A second study found that a large proportion of women with a family history of a first-degree relative with breast cancer and women diagnosed as having breast cancer before age 35 years did not carry germline BRCA1 mutations, nor was there a common family history profile among women who did have BRCA1 germline mutations.[11] If we use the 1994 estimate for approximately 182,000 women who will be diagnosed with breast cancer each year, fewer than 10,000 women will carry the mutated form of BRCA1. Will emphasis on this kind of research bring a reduction in breast cancer to some 172,000 women without the breast cancer gene?

Screening for this gene (indeed, any gene linked to illness) raises implications of enormous social and economic import. If a woman finds that her breast cancer test is positive, will she be denied employment? Denied insurance? The moral and ethical implications don't stop there.

The BRCA1 gene is a suppressor gene, meaning when it is functioning as nature intended, it repairs damage to the DNA of a cell; thus in a way, it acts like a brake on a car. When mutated, the altered gene allows for runaway growth, just as when the brake on a vehicle is disabled, there may be uncontrolled movement. Only the movement, in the case of the altered gene, may be uncontrolled cell growth and spread, that is, cancer.

The Utah-based researchers identified the BRCA1 gene as having five different sites where alterations have occurred. Alterations identified include deletions, an addition, a substitution, an alteration, and a regulatory mutation. Considering that a single gene mutation can result in a loss of a normal body function, five different alterations change not only the structure but the function of that single gene! Considering the number and variety of changes in the suppressor gene, more than likely, not one, but a number of different insults caused these alterations. It is these insults, the causes of the genetic damage, that must be identified.

If you took your smoothly running automobile, deleted half of the spark plugs, added an anchor, substituted one of the wheels with a bicycle wheel, altered the fuel to kerosene, and changed the regulation of the carburetor, your car would not function as intended. The same is true when a few genes are altered.

That the families from whom blood samples were collected lived in Utah raises some interesting questions. Mormon families can be useful for some genetic studies because many keep detailed, long-term genealogical records. According to Dr. Mary-Claire King, blood was collected over a 20-year period beginning in 1976, though she believed that the genetic abnormality existed for a 100 years. In at least one family, the genotype of the grandfather was "deduced," rather than measured.[12]

What were the stimuli that caused the genetic alterations, and when exactly did they begin? By 1976, when the blood collection began, the Utah population had been subjected to fallout from the Nevada test site for 25 years. A total of 26 aboveground tests and 11 underground tests had been detonated between 1951 and 1980, when testing was finally stopped. Dr. Carl Johnson found an excess incidence of cancer (61% for all ages) in Mormon families who lived in southwestern Utah and adjacent areas of Nevada and Arizona throughout the 1951 to 1962 period of bomb testing.[13] By 1996, when the blood collection was complete for the gene identification study, 45 years had passed for cumulative radiation damage to occur.[14] Did the genetic alterations occur over time, to a male or female progenitor, or to both, and when did they originate? We know that in the course of reproduction, each person inherits a copy of each gene from each parent. One gene could be a normal and thus a dominant copy, and the other a defective copy. It is plausible that in the absence of damaging radiation and chemical pollution the gene's protective function would not have been as critical as it is today. What are the insults that the defective copy cannot correct?

Considering the cancer clusters and the BRCA1 were identified in Utah, did the genetic alterations result from various radioactive nucleotides, carried from the Nevada test site, that rained down upon their homes and farms? We do not know if the BRCA1 gene has been present for generations or not. Did the Utah "clan of one-breasted women" suffer genetic damage from radiation as believed by Terry Tempest Williams and so lovingly described in her book *Refuge?*[15] In addition to radiation, what other gene-damaging stimuli were active? Were the insults pesticides, used in homes and on farms, or were they hormones, or hormone-like chemicals, contaminating the food, fish and livestock of the Utah residents?

Two years after I wrote the above paragraph, I was given a copy of a hearing held in 1959. Before we are led to believe that the breast cancer gene is long-inherited, consider the implications of the following, which was known by our Congress: "The genetic injury from both weapon-produced carbon-14 and fission products occurs at the moment the genetic molecule is affected and is the result of absorbed radiation. The actual effect does not appear until this particular gene is found in either the sperm or ovum at the time of fertilization. This event may occur several generations after the initial injury." "Most of the injury due to fission products will be initiated within a 30-year period. By contrast, after the initial transient increase in atmospheric carbon-14 is past, half the remaining carbon-14 injuries will be introduced over a period of 5,600 years, 75 percent in 11,200 years, and so on."[16]

Why is this not well known to the gene researchers? Why is this not well known the bureaucrats at NCI who dole out the money for nearly every research proposal but radiation-induced genetic change? Who was it who said: "If we forget the lessons of history, we are forced to relive them"? Or should the quote end "forced to re-die them?"

Women are already having "prophylactic mastectomies" on the basis of a positive breast cancer gene test. What body part will we next be willing to excise, based upon genetic findings? Now that the nuclear genie is out, how can anyone claim that prophylactic mastectomies are prevention? Isn't primary prevention preferable—that is, to stop chemical pollution, stop nuclear bomb testing, close nuclear power plants, and clean up and control wastes?

What part each or all of these events played in altering the genetic base in BRCA1 is undetermined, and unasked. When in the course of time did these genetic variations appear, and did the genetic mutations occur one at a time or all at once?

The family identified to carry the BRCA1 gene had been found in the Utah Population Database as comprising a group of women with pre-menopausal breast cancer. As if breast cancer were not a sufficient burden, women having an altered BRCA1 gene were linked to a likelihood of developing ovarian cancer as well. The mutation was detected in 3 of 32 women with breast cancer and 1 of 12 women with ovarian cancer.[17]

The researchers collected blood from 195 family members, and collected information from 72 women via questionnaire or through contact with living relatives, recording reproductive history, cancer incidence, treatment, and lifestyle.[18]

The BRCA1 gene, located on a single chromosome, the one designated as 17q, is about 10 times as large as an ordinary gene. Being a large gene, BRCA1 presents a bigger target with more sites to be damaged, and thus altered by insults received in the course of a lifetime. The researchers at the University of Utah, where much of the work was done, found four different mutations in women from the eight families they studied.

For women concerned about the likelihood of developing breast cancer, neither the BRCA1 test nor any other genetic test will be simple or inexpensive. Accurately finding a unique mutation in the mass of the large gene will not be simple. The task of comparing defective genes from different families may prove to be even more elusive. Then, as if this were not a sufficient puzzle, there is the suggestion of two additional genes, BRCA2 and BRCA3, not yet fully identified, and still a third gene, the p53, which is also linked to breast and other cancers. Lastly, some women have variations in their BRCA1 gene and no breast cancer.

Work by biologist Ruth Sager, at the Dana-Faber Cancer Institute in Boston, has identified more than 40 possible tumor-suppressor genes.[19] So it is apparent that a damaged gene, resulting in malignancy, is unique to neither breast cancer nor to the much-touted BRCA genes.

In our technologically oriented society a quick fix is ever anticipated, and prevention ignored. Soon after the initial announcement of the BRCA gene, Ellen Goodman, on the editorial page of the *Washington Post*[20] wrote: "Today we have an answer to a scientific puzzle that comes with a hundred new questions. Just wait until they find the breast cancer gene. Now we wait for the cure." Isn't the bigger challenge to stop the factors damaging our genes?

This hoped-for panacea, a breast cancer gene, is a less bright beacon than touted in the media and by some scientists—anxious to report a "breakthrough." Since gene mutations are multiple, and in differing sites, a single defect (and its single unique cause) will remain undetected. More than likely it is the sum total of various alterations that allow for cell growth to go unchecked. Left unaddressed by genetic research is the question of primary prevention, and the entire task of treatment of those already sick.

How did this breast cancer gene research come about? It was Dr. Mary-Claire King, whose work at the University of California narrowed the location of this particular breast cancer gene to an area of 1000 or so other genes, located in a stretch of DNA on chromosome number-17,[21,22] and it was she who has called for investigation of environmental factors leading to alterations in this gene.

Following Dr. King's lead, Dr. Mark Skolnick and his colleagues at the Utah Medical Center in Salt Lake City used various techniques to isolate the specific gene. Upon submitting the group's findings for publication, Dr. Skolnick said they purposely omitted two critical pieces of information, for fear that the information would get into the hands of the "competition." But no cause for alarm; the crucial sequences had been deposited with GenBank and Myriad Genetics, Inc., a Salt Lake City biotechnology company that applied for a patent and has licensed the use of its genetic knowhow for the development of drugs and diagnostic kits to a subsidiary of Eli Lilly.[23,24] Eli Lilly Corporation is a manufacturer of pharmaceuticals, chemicals, and pesticides. Six of the 45 scientists working on the project were supported by the National Institutes of Health, bringing with them $2 million in federal funds. Eli Lilly contributed another six scientists and $4 million, with product licensing then going to an Eli Lilly subsidiary, Hybritech of San Diego.[25]

One might question the wisdom, ethics, and economics of granting an exclusive patent for a gene technology with such widespread public health implications, especially when the research was supported by tax-derived public money. The director of NIH, Harold Varmus, filed a counterapplication for patent, adding claim for the government-supported NIH scientists to the patent.[26] A settlement was finally reached early in 1995, granting 25% of potential royalties to the U.S. government (read, we the taxpayers). Kept confidential are the terms of the agreement between NIH, the University of Utah, and Myriad Genetics, Inc, thus restricting access to information clearly in the public's interest. Shut out also is the ability of the NIH to set the price of products developed under the patent.[27]

The entire concept of allowing a corporation or any entity to patent human genetic materials has not been resolved. Only France has declared unpatentable "the human body, its elements and products as well as knowledge of the partial or total structure of a human gene."[28] In an encouraging step, a number of scientists from the US., Norway, the Netherlands, and England have formed the International BRCA Consortium (IBC) to share data and laboratory materials regarding breast cancer genes.[29]

Even in the absence of enormous ethical, moral, and economic considerations, impediment to the free flow of information and the assault on human dignity can and should be what stops the patenting of human genetic material.

Granting Eli Lilly a patent on a breast cancer test may be the ultimate irony: Eli Lilly is one of the purveyors of the cancer-causing chemical DES, and until 1997, with Dow Chemical Co. a manufacturer of pesticides, some linked to cancer, neurotoxicity, and hormonal effects. One of Lilly's most financially successful chemicals is their mind-altering drug, Prozac,* perhaps the "soma" of Huxley's *Brave New World*, touted to end our worries and concerns, but paradoxically, linked to tumor promotion. Discussing the effect of Prozac and similar chemicals on cancer growth, a major magazine article leads with "a number of drugs are to cancer as gasoline is to fire."[30]

Other genetic research is controlled by another pharmaceutical/testing giant: SmithKline Beecham, under contractual agreements with The Institute for Genomic Research (TIGR), a nonprofit organization, and with the for-profit corporation, Human Genome Sciences, Inc. (HGS). Each is located in suburban Maryland, close to Washington, D.C.[31] HGS will allow use of its

---

*Prozac (fluoxetine) is distributed by Dista Products Company, a division of Eli Lilly. The label, printed in Physician's Desk Reference, lists 9 columns of information, warnings, and adverse effects concerning the product.

proprietary data, but only after a researcher agrees to allow HGS first option to license any useful products, and only after the researcher grants prior review of any publication.[32] As of 1994, HGS's founder, Craig Venter, held stock in his company valued at $11.5 million.[33]

Within two weeks after the announcement of BRCA1, Eli Lilly announced an 8% increase in its third-quarter net income, to $3187 million, and SmithKline Beecham posted a 4% net increase, to $320 million, for the same period.[34]

A parallel concern arises because SmithKline Beecham owns one of the country's largest clinical laboratory operations. When a physician submits a patient's blood (or any body fluid) sample to a SmithKline Beecham laboratory for analysis, the test results arrive at the physician's office on a computer-generated form. Considering conflicts between commercial and private interests, what safeguards are there that data will not be shared with other business interests? A bill to be sent to the U.S. Congress in 1998 would prohibit American companies from using genetic tests as a basis for firing or for employment benefits, and would bar discrimination against employees with genetic predispositions to a disease.

Will Jane Doe, with a diagnosis of breast cancer, become a "commercial opportunity?" Will commercial exploitation be the least of Jane Doe's worries? Would this very personal (*very, very personal*) and unique information be used against a patient and her children?It takes but little imagination to picture a computer screen with one's genetic information available to anyone with the knowhow to access a data base: insurance companies, employers, persons involved in lawsuits.

Aspects of mankind slated to be tested or altered by genetic manipulation remain unknown outside of the scientists and corporations directing the research with little oversight by the public. While a proposal by National Institutes of Health director Harold Varmus to eliminate the genetics advisory board met with support from the biotechnology industry, opposition by the public ran two to one. A plan to shrink the Recombinant DNA Advisory Committee from 25 to 15 members, without regulatory power, was proposed.[35]

At this time, ethical implications of genetic testing may far outweigh medical benefits Drs. Li and Fraumeni of the National Cancer Institute call for adherence to the four ethical principles of respect: autonomy, beneficence, confidentiality, and justice.[36] Autonomy implies true informed consent and freedom from coercion; beneficence, the time-honored principle of "first do no harm"; confidentiality is straightforward; justice is a tougher issue, requiring freedom from discrimination based upon test results, and full access to health care.

The United States is alone among first-world nations without universal medical care. With some 44 million citizens lacking access to health care, it remains a mystery why the collective public voice does not demand universal, single-payer medical care. Until this is achieved, the medical care industry, as it is currently structured, can and will be allowed to discriminate. Freedom from discrimination and access to patient-oriented health care has become less likely as insurance, corporate medical, and corporate drug interests assume control of medicine extending from basic research to treatment. All of this has been aided and abetted by Congress and well-moneyed political action committees

These critical issues, discussed by the scientific community for some time, go unaddressed by those whose lives are be most affected: current and future patients and their medical personnel. In the interim, control of the issues run full speed into the technological future. Without single-payer medical care for all, the final factor, justice, may be the patient's greatest impediment to using genetic testing.

That genetic research has great commercial potential and significant power is not in dispute. A federal advisory board voted in September 1994 to allow scientists to bypass the NIH approval system and apply directly to the FDA to perform genetic experiments on humans. There is concern that experiments, previously prohibited on ethical grounds, may now be undertaken. Such experiments include alteration of human genes that will be passed on to one's offspring. Under investigation also are some techniques aimed less toward disease amelioration than at cosmetic results, such as manipulating genes to increase a child's height.[37] Media attention to the breast cancer gene—from cover stories in mainstream magazines to articles in scientific journals—brings false hope to many women, and may well cost them considerable money in a futile quest. Lost in the message of the "cancer gene" is the more important fact that the gene is a repair gene. In other words, it is a gene that ought to repair cellular genetic damage, but, because it has been altered, it no longer functions as it was intended.

The prime issue is to identify what factors change a normal gene into a nonfunctional one. If our exposure to toxic chemicals and nuclear radiation were lessened, would the functional ability of protective genes be less critical?

And, shouldn't our financial and scientific priorities be more properly focused in those directions?

If BRCA1 screening becomes an accepted clinical test, then one can propose, on the basis of scientific validity, fairness, and ethical concerns, that dual testing, to assay for foreign, carcinogenic and hormonally active chemicals linked to breast cancer, be done on the same sample. If findings correlate, science will have made a major step in identifying chemicals associated with breast cancer, and thus, a viable step toward prevention.

One expert rightly expressed concern for the cost of a dual, coordinated test. In view of the fact that the manufacturers and polluters that produced many of these hormonally active chemicals are clearly identified, would it not be equitable to place a tax on those corporations to pay for the assays? Such a program would go a long way toward defining the relative roles of genetics and environment: linking the tests makes scientific and economic sense and could end the wrangling and deliberate obfuscation concerning what is a "risk" and what is a cause.

UNCERTAINTIES OF GENETIC TESTING

The announcement of BRCA1 brings questions galore:

- What if a woman finds she is carrying the BRCA1 gene? Can she lessen her chance of developing breast cancer by any means?
- If the woman elects to have a bilateral "prophylactic mastectomy," who will pay the cost?
- For concerned women, would any of the following be useful: Eliminate use of pesticides? Eat a vegetarian diet? Avoid use of birth control pills and post-menopausal hormones? Move away from the vicinity of an incinerator or nuclear reactor? Close the incinerator and nuclear reactor? Don't build an incinerator in the first place? Don't renew the license of a reactor?
- What of the 95%, estimated at 172,000, other women without a genetic predisposition?
- There has to be a cause of this epidemic, and if 95% is not genetic, it must be some other factor we share. What is that factor?
- Is there a link between BRCA1, breast cancer, genital cancer, even prostatic cancer, which is also on the rise?
- If BRCA1 testing is approved, will tests be paid for by insurance companies? By the Federal Government?

- Will the charge for genetic testing be based upon actual cost of development, or will a profit margin be factored in?

- If neither the insurance industry nor the government agrees to pay for such tests, will it mean that poor women and women without insurance will not be afforded the tests?

Until these concerns are answered, we must not allow technology to overwhelm valid scientific, social, ethical, and moral issues. Remembering the words of Martin Luther King, Jr., we may substitute the word genes for the word missiles, but the message remains the same:

> Our scientific power has outrun our spiritual power. We have guided missiles and misguided men.
>
> —*Strength to Love*

REFERENCES

1. Webster's New Universal Unabridged Dictionary. 2nd edition. Simon and Schuster. New York. 1979

2. Breo, D. L. The cancer revolution—from"black box" to"genetic disease." J. Amer. Med. Assoc. 271(18): 1452–1454, 1994.

3. Cover Science. Vol. 266, 1994

4. Hollstein, M., Sidransky, D., Vogelstein, B., Harris, C.C. p53 mutation in human cancers. Science. 253(5015): 49–53, 1991.

5. Aguilar, F., Harris, C.C., Sun, T., Hollstein, M., Cerutti, P. Geographic variation of p53 mutational profile in nonmalignant human liver. Science. 264(5163): 1317–1319, 1994.

6. Chi, Y., Gorina, S., Jeffrey, P.D., Pavletich, N.P. Crystal structure of a p53 tumor suppressor-DNA complex: Understanding tumorigenic mutations. Science. 265: 346–355, 1994.

7. Harris, C.C. p53: At the crossroads of molecular carcinogenesis and risk assessment. Science. 262: 1980–1981, 1993.

8. Miki, Y., and 44 other authors. A strong candidate for the breast and ovarian cancer susceptibility gene BRCA1. Science. 226: 66–71, 1994.

9. Futreal, P.A., and 26 other authors. BRCA1 mutation in primary breast and ovarian carcinomas. Science. 266: 120–122, 1994.

10. Newman, B., Mu, H., Butler, L.M., Millikan, R.C., Moorman, P.G., King, M-C. Frequency of breast cancer attributable to BRCA1 in a population-based series of American women. J. Amer. Med. Assoc. 279(12): 915–921, 1998.

11. Malone, K.E., Daling, J.R., Thompson, J.D., O'Brien, C.A., Francisco, L.V., Ostrander, E.A. BRCA1 mutations and breast cancer in the general

population. J. Amer. Med. Assoc. 279(12): 922–929, 1998.

12. Personal communications. Dr. Mary-Claire King (1-26-95) and Dr. Michelle Bennett (1-18-95).

13. Johnson, C.J. Cancer incidence in an area of radioactive fallout downwind from the Nevada Test Site. J. Amer. Med. Assoc. 251: 230–236, 1984.

14. Johnson, C.J., A cohort study of cancer incidence in Mormon families exposed to nuclear fallout versus an area-based study of cancer deaths in whites in southwestern Utah. Amer. J. Epidemiol. 125(1): 166–168, 1987.

15. Williams, T.T. Refuge: An Unnatural History of Family and Place. Vantage Books, New York. 1991.

16. U.S. 86th Congress Joint Committee on Atomic Energy. Summary-Analysis of Hearings. Fallout from Nuclear Weapons Tests. May 5–8, 1958. p. 28. U.S. Government Printing Office. Washington, D.C. 1959.

17. Futreal et al. Op. cit.

18. Goldgar, D.E., Fields, P., Lewis, C.M., Tran, T.D. A large kindred with 17q-linked breast and ovarian cancer: genetic, phenotypic, and genealogical analysis. J. Nat. Cancer Inst. 86(3): 200–209, 1994.

19. Campbell, A. The science of persistence. Univ. of Chicago. Mag32–35, August 1944.

20. Goodman, E. First the Gene, then the Cure. Washington Post. p. A-15. September 17, 1994.

21. King, M-C. Of mice and women: Genetic analysis of breast cancer in families. Dev. Oncol. 43: 227–236, 1086.

22. Hall, J.M., Lee, M.K., Newman, B., Morrow, J.E., King, M-C. Linkage of early-onset familial breast cancer to chromosome 17Q21. Science. 250(4988): 1684–1689, 1990.

23. Nowak, R. Breast cancer gene offers surprises. Science. 265: 1796–1799, 1994.

24. Weiss, R. Breast cancer gene's impact limited. Washington Post Health. p. 7. September, 20, 1994.

25. Nowak, R. NIH in danger of losing out on BRCA1 patent. Science. 266: 209, 1994.

26. Associated Press. NIH battles over patent on breast cancer gene. Washington Post. p. HV-13. November 1, 1994.

27. Marshall, E. NIH gets a share in BRCA1 patent. Science. 267: 1086, 1995.

28. Knoppers, B.M., Chadwick, R. The human genome project: Under the international ethical microscope. Science. 265: 2035–2036, 1994.

29. Ibid.

30. Brink, S. A different kind of cancer risk. US News & World Report. 58–61, January 9, 1995.

31. Marshall, E. A showdown over gene fragments. Science. 266: 208–210, 1994.

32. Marshall, E. HGS opens its databanks—for a price. Science. 266: 25, 1993.

33. Day, K. Biotech executives find wealth in their genes. Washington Post. p. D-1. April 4, 1994.

34. Anon. Washington Post. p. G-2. October19, 1994.

35. Weiss, R. Compromise would retain but shrink genetic experiments panel. Washington Post p. A-19. November 25, 1996.

36. Li, F.P., Gaber, J.E., Friend, S.H., Strong, L.C., Patenaude, A.F., Juengst, E.T., Reilly, P.R., Correa, P., Fraumeni, J.F., Jr. Recommendations on predictive testing for germ line p53 mutations among cancer-prone individuals. J. Nat. Cancer. Inst. 84(15): 1156–1160, 1992.

37. Weiss, R. Regulations are eased on genetic experiments. Washington Post Health. p. 5. September 20, 1994.

12

THE BREAST CANCER EPIDEMIC ON LONG ISLAND

In this now universal contamination of the environment,
chemicals are the sinister and little recognized partners of radiation
in changing the very nature of the world—the very nature of life.
—Rachel Carson, *Silent Spring*[1]

The old story about the drunk searching beneath a glowing street light for his lost car keys bears retelling. When asked why he wasn't searching across the street, closer to his car, he said "the light is better here." It is becoming clear that much cancer research is conducted in the same way: not necessarily to find anything of significance, but that's where it's easier, and perhaps from the political point of view, safer as well. And of course, that's where the money is.

The Long Island Breast Cancer Study Project (LIBCSP) is a case in point. In the late 1980s, women on Long Island became increasingly aware that their mothers, daughters, sisters, neighbors, and friends were being diagnosed with breast cancer. Asking why, one answer was that the cancers appeared to be occurring in upper socioeconomic Jewish women; that must be the reason. Needless to say this explanation was unsatisfactory to everyone: Jewish, non-Jewish, rich, poor, and middle class. Fortunately, the women came together, formed groups, and pressed for answers, ultimately getting the attention of Congress.

The LIBCSP was initiated by Congress in 1993. The Congressional Act directed the National Cancer Institute (NCI), in cooperation with the National Institute of Environmental Health Sciences (NIEHS), to "conduct a case-control study to assess biological markers of environmental and other potential risk factors contributing to the incidence of breast cancer" in women living on Long Island.[2] Elements of the study were to include:

> "contaminated drinking water, sources of indoor and ambient air pollution, including emissions from aircraft, electromagnetic fields, pesticides and other toxic chemicals, hazardous and municipal waste, and, *such factors as the director determines to be appropriate.*"

To date more than $19,000,000 has been appropriated to this project. The major portion, $7.36 million, has gone to Columbia University. Other players include Sloan-Kettering, that received $4.72 million; two awards totalling $4.28 million to the State University of New York (SUNY) at Stony Brook, Long Island; $1.2 million to the American Health Foundation; and lesser grants to Yale University, the Long Island Jewish Medical Center, and Cold Spring Harbor Laboratory.

In addition to the above main grant recipients, there are 32 subcontractors to the study. Major ones include personnel at Albert Einstein School of Medicine, Mt. Sinai School of Medicine, North Shore University Medical Center, University Medical Center at Stony Brook, Westat, Inc., and Winthrop University Hospital.

Given the way the LIBCSP is organized and being conducted there are serious omissions:

1. Not addressing adverse effects from exposure to chemicals known to have been used on Long Island
2. Not addressing radiation exposures
3. Not addressing the additive and synergistic effects from exposures to multiple chemicals and multiple radiation emissions

Concern about a conflict of interest arose when SUNY Stony Brook, along with Batelle, were awarded a $2 billion, 5-year contract to operate Brookhaven National Laboratory, a major source of radioactive pollution for Long Island.[3] How managers and researchers from SUNY resolved their conflicting interests remains unresolved.

Having so many players in any project has several potential effects: diffusion of responsibility and accountability; increased likelihood of error; and spreading the money thin. It has another, little noticed effect, that which operates so well for such commercial projects as B-2 bombers and nuclear reactors for China: it spreads wide the financial interest to keep a project going, no matter how useless, dangerous, or inept.

A separate $542,997 grant, originally given to Brookhaven National Laboratory, was rescinded. The plan was for scientists at BNL to study the "feasibility of a geographical information system." There was criticism on two counts: BNL is one of the major contaminating facilities on Long Island, raising the question of objectivity; Geographical Integrative System (GIS) techniques have already been demonstrated to be feasible, applicable, useful, and most importantly, already available. Automated systems have been developed to integrate census and topographic information. These can be combined with biological and environmental samples to pinpoint sources of pollution and resultant illnesses. What is more, much of the information is already in the public domain with data available on the internet.

GIS techniques were clearly demonstrated by Colorado State University researcher Dr. Jay Nuckols, at an NCI seminar on the role of GIS-based techniques in cancer studies.[4,5] I later met Dr. Nuckols at his laboratory at Colorado State University in Fort Collins. He demonstrated the GIS process as a "stack of maps" overlain with different information. He showed how GIS methods can combine satellite images; census tract information; historical and current land-use data; location and path of water sources, incinerator and dumps sites; meteorological monitoring; birth, death, and sickness records; and combine them with computer storage programs to make essentially three-dimensional maps.

A less elegant technique of overlaying a map with see-through plastic pages of home sites and illnesses was used by Lois Gibbs and the residents of the Love Canal area and their scientific advisors. Using this technique and filling in data with color markers, Dr. Beverly Paigen and Dr. Marvin Schneiderman found that illnesses followed the path of swales, long covered over, but still transporting toxic chemicals.

The principal investigator for the LIBCSP is epidemiologist Dr. Marilie Gammon. She estimated that approximately 2029 women will be diagnosed to have breast cancer during the 12-month recruitment period. Given an equal number of women to be included as controls, the total number of women in the study will be around 4100, which allots about $4634.15 for each woman.

The enormous cost of the LIBCSP is one factor of concern, but the decision to choose the control women from the Long Island population stretches all scientific credibility. In choosing control groups, whether humans for epidemiological studies or animals for laboratory studies, a control group is selected that does not have the exposure factor(s) under consideration. The stated purpose of the LIBCSP is to determine *what unique factors on Long Island* are resulting in cancer, not what is unique about the women developing cancer. If we live to the ripe old age of 85, one-in-eight of us will develop breast cancer in our lifetime. Given these odds, how can one be assured that of the 2000 control women, 8% or 160 women, don't already have undiagnosed cancer? After all, the control women have lived in the same milieu as the women with cancer.

Since learning of the unconventional choice of a control group, I have asked many different people, with and without scientific training, from where they would choose a control group to compare with Long Island. Without exception, no one chose Long Island. And more than one person remarked, incredulously, "not Long Island?!" But Dr. Gammon and her associates did.

It is true that our world is becoming increasingly contaminated, and as explained by Dr. Steingraber, "there remains no unexposed control population to whom cancer rates of exposed people can be compared. Moreover the exposures themselves are uncontrolled and multiple."[6] Still, why did the NCI-sponsored researchers set up the project this way? As the story unfolds, it will become more clear to the reader, as it has to many Long Island women, that the LIBCSP has serious, if not fatal, flaws.

The LIBCSP is conducted as a case-control study, that is, choosing a person without breast cancer to match with a woman who has breast cancer, taking into consideration such factors as age, race, etc. A case-control study is one of the most blunt of research instruments, especially given the way this one is being conducted, with cases and controls living in the same area. Given the same level of funding, if the inappropriately chosen control subjects were not included, there would be over $9000 to do thorough biological and environmental testing for each and every woman with breast cancer.

Another issue of concern is who is eligible to be in the study. The study defines the participants as women "newly diagnosed with primary breast cancer, and whose physician has given consent for contact."[7] Some women feel that this arrangement was condescending and controlling, and wonder why the women were not recruited directly. There are 136 participating physicians, making patient enrollment cumbersome, variable, and incomplete.

The study design expects 1623 cases and the same number of controls to be interviewed. Of these, 60% "are expected to provide biological specimens," and approximately 325 of each group (650 total) who have resided 15 years or longer in their current residence will have home assessments of dust, drinking water, and soil. Of the 974 women with cancer (60% of 1623) who provide blood and urine specimens, fewer than half of the samples will be analyzed, the rest "banked for future use."[8]

The Long Island women have expressed serious concerns over the handling of blood samples: insufficient quantities drawn; clotting of some samples; lack of coordination with environmental sampling; and samples obtained from women after radiation and/or chemotherapy treatment had begun. This last issue, comparing biological data from women without cancer to biological data obtained from women undergoing cancer treatment, is folly, and questionable science at best.

More numbers, and the numbers tell the story: 60% of the total number of women interviewed equals 1951, and 650 women are to have three different environmental assays, for a total of 1950 assays or a grand total of approximately 3900 biological and environmental samples to be analyzed.

The following is a direct quote as of December 1996: "That of the 650 participants (325 cases and 325 controls) with environmental samples, approximately 60 percent ($n = 390$) will have donated blood and urine specimens. Of that 390 (175 invasive cancer cases, 20 in situ cases, and 195 controls), about 40 percent ($n = 148$); 70 invasive cases and 78 controls) will be randomly selected for the lab assays of their blood and urine."[9]

Those are confusing numbers to comprehend, but if the numbers are correct, of some 1600 women who develop breast cancer during the period of study, roughly 4% can expect to have a full assay of both biological and environmental samples. Stated another way, after the expenditure of all the money, time, and effort, 96% of women will have no meaningful information. For the rest of the participants, the study design gives no assurance that biological and environmental samples will be taken from the *same* woman.

Review of the "Results" portion of the "Background" document of Dr. Marilie Gammon's part of the study reveals another interesting point of view: the very narrow approach taken to the issue of cancer-causing chemicals, limiting the categories to "possible human breast carcinogens" and further limiting the list to DDT, DDE, PCBs, and chlordane.[10] Moreover, there is no provision to assay body fat samples for suspect chemicals.

Aside from being chlorinated organic chemicals with known toxic effects, what do these chemicals have in common? These named chemicals have already been banned! That means no corporate entity will be embarrassed and on-the-line to stop production of any of the products in the United States. It also means that other carcinogenic and hormonally active chemicals, known to have been used on Long Island, are not under scrutiny in the Long Island breast cancer epidemic.

Citing lack of funds to include chemicals other than DDT, DDE, PCBs, and chlordane poses the question of whether this decision was to avoid offending a chemical manufacturer, supplier, or user of other candidate chemicals. Given that breast cancer is not the only cancer or the only serious medical problem on Long Island, this restricted view suggests a certain lack of perspective about connections between environmental factors, endocrine disruption, birth defects, other cancers, and other illnesses.

The scientific literature survey given in the "Background" document[11] shows a paucity of sources and a remarkable lack of historical information about chemical pesticides known to have been used on Long Island. Until the early 1970s there were 80,000 to 100,000 acres of potatoes grown on Long Island. Suffolk County was the third largest potato grower in the world, behind Maine and Idaho. Because of fear of a Colorado potato beetle infestation, pesticides were sprayed as often as every 10 days, from May to August. This was told to me by Dr. Robert Simon, who himself did spraying, applying Temik (aldicarb), dieldrin, endrin, chlordane, parathion, and DDT.[12]

Adding to Long Island's toxic chemical load were PCBs, which Dr. Simon related to have migrated from multiple sites, the major contributor being the General Electric (GE) plants near Fort Edwards and Hudson Falls, New York.[13] By 1977, GE estimated there were 137 metric tons of PCBs on the river's floor,[14] which has led to advisories against eating fish from the river.[15] Flowing southward along the east border of New York state, the Hudson River is deceptively beautiful as it passes the state capital in Albany, the Roosevelt and Vanderbilt estates near Hyde Park, and further south, the West Point Military Academy. Near its mouth, the river flows by the west side of Manhattan and the borough of Brooklyn, which makes up the western end of Long Island.

So contaminated is the river that the federal government has designated the entire stretch of the Hudson River, downstream from the GE plant to New York Harbor, as a Superfund site![16]

In addition to exposures from contaminated water and soil is the potential for even wider exposure as a result of air dispersion of PCBs. Citizens have voiced concern that delays in addressing the contamination may have played a factor in the transfer of Department of Health researcher Dr. Brian Bush. Dr. Bush had been with the New York research post for 25 years when he was told to "cease PCB analyses" immediately.[17]

In support of their decision to eliminate DBCP, toxaphene, and styrene from testing, the Columbia researchers cited as "the most comprehensive source of information"[18] documents prepared by subcontractors of Agency for Toxic Substances and Disease Registry (ATSDR) some time before 1990.[19–21] By and large, ATSDR documents are not historical compendia, but reviews of relatively recent publications. The most recent citation in the styrene document was 1989, but even that publication cited three studies that were positive for mammary cancer in test animals.[22] Dibromochloropropane (DBCP) is a soil "sterilant" and is widely used in agriculture. Though now banned in the United States, DBCP remains detectable in the water supply of many communities. So far, this issue has been ignored.[23]

Dr. Gammon's memo that "no meaningful data has [sic] been published with regard to the carcinogenicity of methoxychlor," and regarding 2,4-D and 2,4,5-T, "there is insufficient evidence to conclude that they are human carcinogens"[24] escapes credibility. The components of Agent Orange, 2,4-dichlorophenoxyacetic acid (2,4-D) and 2,4,5-trichlorophenoxyacetic acid (2,4,5-T), were used extensively in agriculture, and while 2,4,5-T has been largely banned in the United States, 2,4-D remains in common use on lawns and golf courses. Methoxychlor is similar in structure to DDT and is documented to be carcinogenic.[25] Criticism of ATSDR and its methods has been documented in the publication *Inconclusive by Design*, the last citation in this chapter.

Long Island women have requested that dioxins be included in the assays because of known carcinogenicity and endocrine disruption and the high probability that dioxins, as well as the carcinogen cadmium, are emitted from incinerators located on Long Island. To date this valid request has not been done.

The considerable data on endocrine disruption, researched by Dr. Theo Colborn[26] and her associates, applicable to the cancer problem for the chemicals 2,4-D, 2,4,5-T, atrazine, atrazine, endosulfan, and alkyphenols, were dismissed with the statement "no meaningful data exists [sic] in regard to their carcinogenicity, either in humans or animals."[27] And so, these chemicals, along with the phthalates and aldicarb also will not be looked for.

Why the decision was made not to assay for other chemicals is not known. One would expect that simple curiosity would have driven a broader perspective. The women activists proposed more thorough chemical testing. In response to their proposals, the researchers labeled their requests a "wish list," a condescending and dismissive reply to their legitimate concerns.

The soil-sampling plan and soil assay for polycyclic aromatic hydrocarbons (PAH) and nitro-PAH also pose problems for the LIBCSP participants. The original idea was to collect a single soil sample. Because this was inadequate, the protocol was expanded to collect four samples—two samples from the yard, and two obtained within 15 inches or less from the house foundation. The latter is thought to be where chemicals accumulate: chemicals such as paint components, termite and other pesticide treatments, and rainborne chemicals from roof runoff. The soil protocol says analysis "will be carried out on every fourth sample received, the remainder being stored frozen for later analysis if and when funds become available."[28] The protocol does not state which "every fourth sample" will be analyzed. Will it be a sample from close to a house, from the yard, where?

The soil collection data form asks for information on herbicide and pesticide use, but the protocol does not include analysis for herbicides and pesticides. No other assays are indicated, other than for polycyclic aromatic hydrocarbons, the PAHs, and their nitrated relatives, the N-PAHs.

The entire soil assay problem begins with the method for collecting the soil. The protocol is illuminating. It says to put each soil sample into a plastic baggie, with a preprinted self-adhesive label, put two rubber bands around the baggie, and "place the four baggies next to each other, and band them together as well. Place the four banded baggies inside a larger zip-lock bag" with a pink laboratory copy form inside the last bag. The soil samples are then to be shipped with a frozen cold pack inside another baggie, with newspaper stuffed inside the packing box. Furthermore, the protocol states that if Federal Express is closed, to keep the samples "in your refrigerator or cooler."

Think about the above. Plastics leach into samples, samples decrease in amounts as they leach into plastics, rubber bands are made of chemicals, self-stick labels are manufactured with chemical glues, newspaper ink has solvents and other chemicals, the samples can be stored in a home refrigerator, and we don't even know what's inside the cold pack! Is this any way to conduct research? I've checked my own knowledge of soil chemistry with two industrial hygienists, and the word is *glass*. Yes, as with blood and urine samples, soil samples must be collected and stored in *tightly sealed glass* to maintain integrity of the samples and to avoid cross-contamination.

Why was this not known by officials at NCI and Columbia University and by the people at American Health Foundation, where the assays are to be done?

The carcinogenic effects from exposure to polynuclear aromatic hydrocarbons (also called PAH's) have been known for decades.[29] These chemicals are released from incinerators and various industrial operations.[30] One such PAH is methylcholanthrene, having both estrogenic and carcinogenic properties. When combined with x-ray exposure, PAHs caused leukemia in several strains of mice.[31] On Long Island, such combined exposures, involving multiple chemicals and nuclear radiation, is a reality. Why is this situation not being addressed by the NCI-sponsored study?

A portion of the LIBCSP that follows sound scientific methodology and procedure is the work of Drs. Bradlow and Kabat. Previous work by Drs. Bradlow and Davis has demonstrated an increased risk for breast cancer with alteration of the ration between 16-alpha- and 2-hydroxyestrone, the metabolites of estrogens.[32] Dr. Bradlow's group is researching several common pesticides that appear to increase production of the 16-alpha-hydroxysterone as a link to breast cancer. It is likely that research directed to this problem may produce some valid and useful results.

Of the many shortcomings of the LIBCSP, perhaps the most serious is the failure to collect data on nuclear radiation as a factor in the Long Island breast cancer epidemic. Extensive research links low-level radiation, alone and combined with chemical exposure, to cancer.

Unequivocally, Long Island is a place with a history of toxic chemical and radiation releases. In addition to the Brookhaven National Laboratory and its nuclear facility, Long Island is in close proximity to the Millstone and Haddam Neck reactors in Connecticut; the Indian Point reactor in Peekskill; and downwind from New Jersey's Oyster Creek reactor. Perhaps it is too much for citizens to expect million dollar governmental-sponsored multisite studies to provide either information or prevention.

A case in point is the small, independent research group, Radiation and Public Health Project, Inc. (RPHP) headed by Dr. Jay Gould. Data collected by RPHP concerning radiation nationwide can be found on the internet at www.radiation.org.

Dr. Gould and his associates accessed information from the New York Health Department's Statewide Planning and Resource Cooperative System (SPARCS). When they analyzed data for hospital discharges for breast malignancy for Suffolk County, the home of Brookhaven National Laboratory, they found that for the 1990 Suffolk population of 692,000 women, the rate of breast cancer for the county was 1.99 cases per 1000. This was somewhat higher than the corresponding rate of 1.91 cases per 1000 in

New York City, and the nationwide rate of 1.7. In five zip code areas representing parts of five towns surrounding BNL, the breast cancer rate was 3.64 cases per 1000 population They calculated that more than half of the female population of Suffolk county lives within a 20-mile radius of BNL. By dividing the circle into quadrants, they were able to add three other zones east and west of the circle to display the full variation in cancer discharges. The highest breast cancer rate (4.0 per 1000) is found in women living on the north fork of Peconic Bay, downstream from BNL and only 11 miles downwind from the troubled Millstone nuclear reactors.[33]

To coordinate the findings of cancer and nuclear pollution in areas of Long Island and elsewhere, as Toms River, New Jersey, the RPHP has initiated the "Tooth Fairy Project" to collect baby teeth for measurement of strontium 90. By calling 1-800-582-3716, parents, teachers, and public health personnel can get instructions on how to send baby teeth for analysis. Perhaps the most critical aspect of the study is the realization that measuring levels of radionuclides in baby teeth gives irrefutable clinical and geographic evidence of prior contamination.

As if radiation pollution were not of sufficient concern, a 1996 survey of Peconic River silt found mercury and silver at levels more than 1000 times the criteria for the New York State Department of Environmental Conservation. Copper and lead were detected in seven of 12 samples of fish, and DDD, a metabolite of DDT and the PCB Aroclor-1254, was found in all four fish that were sampled. Additionally, tritium and cesium 137 were found in all three samples analyzed for radionuclides.[34] A 1998 survey of fish from the Peconic River, both on- and off-site of the BNL property, found lead, mercury, nickel; the DDT metabolites DDE and DDT; and strontium 90 and cesium 137 in nearly all fish samples.[35]

A New York Department of Health document calculated radiation doses for those who consumed fish, clams, or mussels harvested from Peconic River waters. "Due to the long residence within the body of Sr 90 and Cs 137, the radiation dose is delivered to body tissue over a long period of time [some 50 years] following ingestion."[36]

These findings were reported in the press throughout 1997 and 1998. Groundwater from BNL was contaminated with plutonium, uranium, americium, strontium, and cesium; tritium had been released into the air;[37] plutonium from BNL had infiltrated the Peconic River,[38] with measurable quantities 1 mile from the laboratory;[39] and in 1996, radioactive cesium had been measured in deer living near the site.[40]

Given the many surveys and historical data that have demonstrated significant chemical and radiological pollution on Long Island, and the avowed purpose of the NCI-led LIBCSP to specifically address environmental factors contributing to the high incidence of breast cancer on Long Island, the result of the research may be that the LIBCSP will not find any connection between breast cancer and the environment. With its narrow, unimaginative approach, it appears it may discover little else of interest as well.

Many on Long Island ask why research into factors causing breast cancer in Long Island women, as done by the NCI-sponsored, Columbia-led research, is being conducted in such an unfocused and incomplete manner. They ask too when all the time, money, and effort have been exhausted, will the LIBCSP be another example of *"Inconclusive by Design?"*[41]

REFERENCES

1. Carson, R. Silent Spring. Crest Books. New York. p. 16, 1962.
2. Public Law 103-43, June 10, 1993, Section 1911.
3. Lawler, A. SUNY-Batelle team to run Brookhaven. Science. 278: 1702, 1997.
4. Nuckols, J. National Cancer Institute seminar, held March 7, 1996.
5. Nuckols, J.R. Use of remote sensing technology in a health assessment of rural agricultural communities. Amer. Inst. Aeronautics and Astronautics. pp. 1–10. 1995.
6. Steingraber, S. Living Downstream. Addison Wesley. Reading, MA. p. 29. 1997.
7. Gammon, M., Neuget, A., Santella, R. Long Island Breast Cancer Study Project. Columbia University Case-Control Study. 6 pages. No date.
8. Gammon et al. Op. Cit.
9. Gammon, M. D. LIBCSP. Year 2 Progress Report Summary. December 1996.
10. Gammon, M. "Background" document. pp. 1–14. No date.
11. Gammon, M. Op. Cit.
12. Simon, R. Telephone interview. September 24, 1997.
13. Sack. K. G. E. To stop flow of PCBs into the Hudson River. New York Times. p. 38. July 18, 1993.
14. Sullivan, W. G.E., whose plants spilled PCBs, sees signs of natural breakdown. New York Times. p. 18. June 9, 1987.
15. Gold, A. R. After 15 years, Hudson still has PCBs. New York Times. p. B-1. May 16, 1990.
16. Rivlin, M. A. Muddy Waters: GE, PR and PCBs. Amicus J. 19(4): 30–37, 1997.
17. Anon. Poughkeepsie Journal. N. Y. forces scientist to stop work on PCB-health link. p. 1-A. September, 27, 1997.
18. Gammon, M. Op. Cit.
19. ATSDR. Toxicological Profile for 1,2-dibromo-3-chloropropane. Prepared by

Syracuse Research corporation, under subcontract to: Clement Associates, Inc. 1990.

20. ATSDR. Toxicological Profile for Toxaphene. Prepared by Clement Associates. 1990.

21. ATSDR. Toxicological Profile for Styrene. Prepared by Life Systems, Inc., under subcontract to: Clement Associates, Inc. 1990.

22. Gammon, M. Op. Cit.

23. Allen, R. H., Gottlieb, M., Clute, E., Pongsiri, M. J., Sherman, J. D., Obrams, G. I. Breast cancer and pesticides in Hawaii: The need for further study. Environ. Health Perspect. 105(3): 679–683, 1997.

24. Gammon, M. D. Memo to: Community Activists Request for a "Wish List" for the LIBCSP. April 24, 1997.

25. Sherman, J. D. Structure-activity relationships of chemicals causing endocrine, reproductive, neurotoxic, and oncogenic effects—A public health problem. Toxicol. Indust. Health. 10(3): 163–179, 1994.

26. Colborn, T., Clement, C., Eds. Chemically-Induced Alterations in Sexual and Functional Development: The Wildlife/ Human Connection. Princeton Scientific Publishing Co., Inc. 403 pages. 1992.

27. Gammon, M. Op. Cit.

28. Beyea, J., Hatch, M., Grimson, R., Stellman, S., Gammon, M. Draft of soil sampling protocol. 8 pages. January 8, 1997.

29. Lee, S. D., Grant, L., Editors. Health and Ecological Assessment of Polynuclear Aromatic Hydrocarbons. J. Environ. Pathol. Toxicol. 5(1): 1–376, 1981.

30. Santodonato, J., Howard, P., Basu, D. Health and Ecological Assessment of Polycyclic Aromatic Hydrocarbons. J. Environ. Pathol. Toxicol. 5(1): 1–364, 1981.

31. Kirschbaum, A., Shapiro, J. R., Mixer, H. W. Induction of leukemia in mice by estrogenic hormone, methylcholanthrene and x-rays. Cancer Res. 12: 275, 1952.

32. Davis, D. L., Bradlow, H. L. Can environmental estrogens cause breast cancer? Sci. Amer. 166–172, October 1995.

33. Gould, J. M. Radiation and Public Health Project, Inc. April, 1998.

34. IT Corporation. Operable unit V—Fish tissue bioaccumulation study report. Submitted to Brookhaven National Laboratory Associated Universities, Inc. BLN Contract No. 710617. December 9, 1996.

35. IT Corporation. Operable Unit V—Additional fish bioaccumulation study report. Submitted to Brookhaven National Laboratory Associated Universities, Inc. BLN Contract No. 710617. May 27, 1998.

36. New York State Department of Health, Bureau of Environmental Radiation Protection. Radioactive Contamination in the Peconic River. p. 7. September 12, 1996.

37. Pleven, L. Isotopes in lab water. Newsday. p. A-1. October 24, 1997.

38. Rau, J. Calls to widen pollution probe: Plutonium spurs push for Peconic cleanup. Newsday. p. A-1. June 17, 1998.

39. Rau. J., Zehren, C. Plutonium in Peconic River. Newsday. p. A-1. June 11, 1998.

40. Rau, J., Cesium is found in deer at BNL. Newsday. p. A-6. April 30, 1998.
41. Environmental Health Network and National Toxics Campaign Fund. Inconclusive By Design—Waste, Fraud and Abuse in Federal Environmental Health Research. P. O. Box 16267, Chesapeake, VA 23328-6267.

13

DISEASES IN MEN
BREAST, PROSTATE, AND TESTICULAR CANCER, AND SPERM ABNORMALITIES

We are our brothers keepers too.

In keeping with our increasingly polluted environment, it is now more common for men, along with women, to be diagnosed with breast cancer. The threats to life cut across the sexes, the miles, species, and centuries.

CANCER IN HISTORY

It was in males that the link between exposure to chemicals and cancer was first established. This observation occurred over 200 years ago, when in England, Sir Percival Pott described cancer of the scrotum in chimney sweeps.[1] These victims were the poor, undernourished, small, young men and who did the dirty work of cleaning the insides of chimneys. The chemicals, clinging to the folds of their skin, induced cancers that spread through their genitalia into their abdomens, killing them.[2]

While scrotal cancer is no longer common, due in part to fewer chimneys to be cleaned and better access to soap and water, the products of combustion, the soot, tars, stilbenes, and polycyclic organic chemicals, are still a part of our environment and are still factors in the continuing cancer epidemic.

MALE BREAST CANCER

Men are learning that breast cancer is not exclusively a woman's disease. Until recently, men's involvement in breast cancer has been largely as supporters of wives, mothers, and daughters as they battle the surgical, medical, and psychological burdens of the dreaded diagnosis. Now, more men are learning they too have breast cancer.

Increasingly, young boys are developing breast enlargement. A reader's inquiry about the problem to the Health Section of the *Washington Post* was answered by suggesting that the boy with breast enlargement take a drug such as tamoxifen or clomiphene, the latter a fertility drug. In response to the inquiry, no exploration of factors causing breast enlargement for the boy was offered. A boy with breast enlargement should have a thorough medical evaluation and should include inquiry into perinatal as well as subsequent exposure factors. The medical history should include diet, such as meat and dairy products, that may contain growth agents, and whether the child received a significant exposure to estrogenic hormones prior to birth.

What lies ahead for these boys remains uncertain, for there is no registry to follow them. It would be prudent to obtain blood or fat samples for assay of chemicals known to have estrogenic effects. Will the boys who develop breast enlargement be the ones who later develop breast cancer? Will these boys have impaired fertility? These are issues ripe for study.

The work of the Danish pediatric endocrinologist Niels Skakkebaek is of sufficient importance to the public to covered in the popular press. In researching endocrine-related abnormalities in young boys, Dr. Skakkebaek learned that many hormonal products are used as growth agents in livestock, and that dairy cows are often milked while they are still in calf, the period of time when hormones levels are high.[4]

A newspaper story of a 38-year-old man with breast cancer raises troubling questions.[5] After undergoing mastectomy, radiation, and chemotherapy, he was placed on tamoxifen. Within 3 weeks of taking the drug, he reported a 20-pound weight gain. Considering that tamoxifen is not directly anticarcinogenic, but has both estrogenic and antiestrogenic properties, is it an appropriate drug to give to a man?[6]

Of some 180,200 persons diagnosed with breast cancer this year, approximately 1400 are men. Given that breast cancer is unusual in men, the male patients are an optimal group from whom to obtain full environmental and occupational assessments, and to do comprehensive fat assays for xenobiotic chemicals. Unfortunately, there is no known program in place.

In 1980, I examined R.F., a 37-year-old man who had been diagnosed with breast cancer a year earlier. R.F. had worked in a tire manufacturing plant, where he was exposed to multiple chemicals, many carcinogenic and hormonally active. Although two of his coworkers had developed cancer—

one with kidney cancer, the other with metastatic malignant melanoma—it was R.F. whose cancer site was the most uncommon. The carcinogenic hazards of the rubber industry are well characterized in a publication released nearly two decades ago by the International Agency for Research in Cancer.[7] My own research on chemicals used in rubber manufacture revealed that stilbenes were a part of that chemical stew. Significantly, the biologically active stilbenes[8] form the backbone of such products as stilbestrol, tamoxifen, and clomiphene.

Why should this be a surprise? Over a half-century ago, the link between stilbestrol and cancer was well established, producing testicular cancers in mice.[9] And earlier than that, the discoverer of diethylstilbestrol (DES), found low-order estrogenic properties in extracts of "peat, brown coal, lignite, coal-tar, and petroleum,"[10] as well as both estrogenic and carcinogenic properties in several polycyclic aromatic hydrocarbon chemicals (PAH).[11] These findings are pertinent to both men and women, exposed as we are to these biologically active chemicals in our environment, work places, and food supply.

PROSTATE CANCER

Prostate cancer, like breast cancer, is also not an uncommon disease. In 1997, it was estimated that 317,000 men would be diagnosed with the disease and that 48,000 would die from it, affecting black males in greater numbers than their white brothers. Prostatic cancer has been to linked a variety of factors, including occupational exposure to cadmium, found in metal operations, some paint pigments, and welding.[12] Comparing areas with particulate air pollution, the mortality rate for prostatic cancer was 2.7 times higher in the most polluted zone, as compared to areas with fewer particulates.[13] A study of 15,000 white men found that those with a relatively elevated growth factor (IGF-1) in their blood were 4 times as likely to develop prostate cancer, furthering the concerns over the use of IGF-1 stimulating growth hormone (rBGH) in dairy cows.[14] It has been asked: "If little boys drink milk from rBGH-treated cows over long periods, will the elevated levels of IGF-1 increase their prostate cancer rates?"[15] The number of men affected with prostate cancer approaches the incidence of women with breast cancer, and the environmental links may well be the same: chemical carcinogens, endocrine disrupters, and radiation. In a recent study, Dr. Jay Gould utilized data from the Connecticut Cancer registry that, in 1945 before the onset of the nuclear age, was the only registry to keep records. He found that for men aged 50 to 74, the age-adjusted death rate from prostate cancer increased in the years from 1952–1956, during the time of aboveground nuclear testing.[16] With cessation of the tests in 1963, the death rate leveled off until 1971. In the 22 years between 1971 to 1992, deaths increased from 20 to 27 per 100,000 men. More strikingly, in that same period, the incidence of prostate cancer per 100,000 men rose from 100 to 400. While some of the increase may be due in part to improved diagnostic methods, it remains that the increase is real.

Using Freedom of Information requests, Dr. Gould and his colleague, Joseph Mangano, obtained raw data from the National Cancer Institute's large data base, maintained since 1950 and arranged by state for some 3000 counties. They were able to calculate age-adjusted death rates for prostate cancer across the United States. They compared rates from 1985–89 with those of 1950–54 for 14 counties that were within a 50- to 100-mile radius of six major nuclear facilities. These facilities were located in Hanford, Washington; Oak Ridge, Tennessee; Idaho National Engineering, Idaho; Savannah River, bordering on Georgia and South Carolina; Los Alamos, Sandia, in New Mexico; and Brookhaven on Long Island in New York state. Over that time span, while death rates across the United States increased from 15.8 to 16.3 per 100,000 men, the rate for those 14 counties increased from 14.9 to 17.8 per 100,000. More simply said, for the time period from 1950–54 to 1985–89 the prostate cancer death rate increased across the United Sates by 3%, while in the 14 counties with nuclear facilities, the increase was 19%. But it is not just this analysis that is important.

The greater significance lies in the fact that the NCI data base was collected from every state department of health at a cost of billions of dollars, but never before published and made available to the public. Additional information, including tables with specific prostate cancer rates, arranged by state and county will soon be published in full and made available to all.[17]

A Prostate Cancer Prevention Trial (PCPT) has been proposed by the NCI, utilizing the anti-androgen drug finasteride. The plan is to enroll 18,000 men at 220 medical centers over a 10-year period to test finasteride against a placebo. Finasteride, known commercially as Proscar, is manufactured by Merck and acts to lower the hormone 5-alpha-dihydrotestosterone (DHT) via blocking the enzyme that converts testosterone to DHT. It is thought that both noncancerous and cancerous enlargement of the prostate may be controlled by this drug. It is unknown how many men will participate in such a prevention trial. A warning on the use of finasteride states:

> It is not known whether the amount of finasteride that could potentially be absorbed by a pregnant women through either direct contact with crushed Proscar tablets or from the semen of a patient taking Proscar can adversely affect a developing male fetus. . . . Therefore because of the potential risk to a male fetus, a woman who is pregnant or who may become pregnant should not handle crushed Proscar tablets; in addition, when the patient's sexual partner is or may become pregnant, the patient should either avoid exposure of his partner to semen or he should discontinue Proscar.[18]

Adverse effects in rats exposed in utero to finasteride included hypospadias (a split in the surface of the penis) in up to 100% of the offspring, decreased prostatic and seminal vesicular weights, and transient nipple development.[19]

In contrast to the thousands of women who allowed themselves to be recruited into the tamoxifen "prevention" breast cancer study, the study jointly run by the Department of Veteran's Affairs and the National Cancer Institute to determine optimal treatment for men with prostate cancer, could not recruit a single volunteer at several centers, and found only 315 men at the Minnesota Veteran's medical center.[20] The professed reasons were that the men did not want another person making decisions for them.

TESTICULAR DYSFUNCTION, MALFORMATIONS, AND CANCER

Environmental estrogens have been implicated in declining sperm counts worldwide.[21] Analysis of 14,947 men included in 61 papers published between 1938 and 1991 showed a significant decrease in both sperm count and seminal fluid volume. The authors discuss the significance of hormonal dysfunction with concomitant increase in testicular cancer, undescended testicles, and abnormalities of the penis.[22] Congenital malformations of the genitalia were 3 times more common in men exposed in utero to DES than men in a control group.[23] The timing of exposures to environmental factors resulting in sperm decline may be as critical as the chemicals themselves. One must consider exposures occurring during prenatal life as well as subsequent exposures from the diet, the environment, and ones' occupation.

Between 1968 and 1993, the incidence of hypospadias doubled in the United States.[24] Nine to 12 weeks after conception, as the male develops inside the womb, the urethra, a channel for urine, develops in the penis. Failure of this channel to close results in an open channel on the underside of the penis, which may extend all the way to the scrotum.

Genital, central nervous system, facial, and other defects in children exposed before birth to the pesticide chlorpyrifos have been reported.[25–27] The defects are similar to those produced in test animals exposed to chlorpyrifos, a chlorinated organophosphate, and to trichloropyridinol, its metabolic breakdown component.[28–31]

The incidence of testicular cancer is ominous. An extensive study of this disease in six European countries demonstrates an increase in testicular cancer in males born after 1920, leveling off during the years of the Second World War in Denmark, Norway, and Sweden, and increasing again in men born after 1945 in all six countries. These findings are indicative of environmental factors, particularly chemicals carried in the food supply. "Diet" is often cited as the cause of a panoply of non-tobacco-related cancers, but the proponents of this theory fail to note that fat-containing foods are the carriers of fat-soluble toxic chemicals as well as nearly all radionuclides. During times of war, it is the meat, butter, and oils that are in short supply, shifting the food supply to grains and legumes. By 1965, compared to men born in 1905, the relative risk of developing testicular cancer had increased over baseline to 3.9 in Sweden and to 11.4 in the East German Democratic Republic.[32]

A previous study of the these six countries, plus the Baltic countries of Estonia, Latvia, and Lithuania, found similar increases.[33] That such a wide area was under consideration—Estonia, Latvia, Lithuania, Denmark, Norway, Sweden, East Germany, Finland, and Poland, all within the chemically and radiologically polluted Baltic and North Atlantic area—makes it impossible to dismiss the implications and significance of such findings.

Although testicular cancer accounts for fewer than 1% of all male cancer deaths, it accounts for 11 to 13% of deaths for males between the ages of 15 and 34. Even these statistics do not reveal the full extent of the problem, because testicular cancer, relatively easy to detect at an early stage, has a high cure rate. The incidence of testicular cancer doubled between 1937 and 1971, and is still increasing. Occupations specifically linked to testicular cancer are in agriculture, and oil and gas extraction.[34] Testicular cancer in a group of aircraft repairmen[35] and in tannery workers[36] was hypothesized to have been caused by exposure to dimethylforamide, a chemical used in such work.

A conference held by the European Environment Agency (EEA) in December 1996 brought together governmental and chemical industry organizations to address chemical pollution and reproductive disorders.[37] The conclusions of the EEA conference[38] and those from a previous conference held by Theo Colborn and her associates[39] bear attention and action. Spread across the globe are ominous findings for not only the human, but for the male of many species:

- Male fish have produced vitellogenin, a protein found normally only in females.
- Turtles and alligators have been identified with reduced ability to mate due to abnormally small penises.
- Female snails and mussels, exposed to endocrine-disrupting chemicals, have transformed into males.
- Laboratory rats and hamsters, exposed to dioxins shortly before and after birth have reduced sperm counts.
- Rats exposed to PCBs prior to birth have disturbed thyroid function,and as a side-effect have small testicles and reduced sperm counts as adults.
- Early puberty has been produced in rats exposed to PCBs prior to birth.
- Birth defects of the penis (hypospadias) and undescended testicles have been produced in male rodents exposed to endocrine disrupting chemicals.

The EEA report specifically associates adverse effects in rodents with exposure to the pesticide Vinclozolin, patented in 1973 by BASF.[40] In the United States, this fungicide with powerful antiandrogenic properties can be used on cucumbers, grapes, lettuce, onions, bell peppers, raspberries, strawberries, tomatoes, Belgian endive, and turf grasses.[41]

Describing how vinclozolin interferes with androgen-mediated sex development, as well as interference by DDT and DDE, the authors state: "Environmental chemicals with anti-androgenic activity offer profound implications with regard to recent clinical observations that suggest an increasing incidence of human male genital malformations, male infertility, and female breast cancer."[42] Three years earlier, researchers from this same laboratory found that pregnant rats, given vinclozolin, gave birth to males with abnormal genitalia. Findings included small and cleft penises, abnormal and undescended testicles, vaginal (female) pouches, atrophic seminal vesicles, and abnormally placed prostate glands.[43,44] These researchers are from the Reproductive Toxicology Division of the U.S. EPA, the same agency that registers the use of vinclozolin. One must question why this product is on the market. Vinclozolin is but one pesticide registered by the

U.S. EPA that has been found to have adverse effects upon reproduction and/or is a cause of cancer.

The problems of pesticide registration in the United States have been well documented by Dr. John Wargo, in his book *Our Children's Toxic Legacy— How Science and Law Fail to Protect Us from Pesticides*.[45] Citing EPA examples that have failed to protect the health of United States citizens, he notes lesser developed countries lack even those provisions. In light of what is known about adverse effects, complacency seems to rule. There has been no march on the EPA or on Congress to err on the side of public safety.

Abnormal sperm are found in farm workers who sprayed the herbicide 2,4-dichlorophenoxyacetic acid (2,4-D), resulting in both dead and abnormal sperm forms, raising the specter of birth defects in children conceived when these surviving sperm are active.[46] 2,4-D is a weedkiller, commonly used on lawns, golf courses, and in agriculture. When mixed with the nearly identical chemical, containing one more chlorine atom, it becomes Agent Orange, the herbicide sprayed over Vietnam.

The use of chemicals with carcinogenic, sperm-damaging, antimale hormone actions on lawns, golf courses, and playing fields ought to give pause for anyone, child or adult. The joys and health benefits from exercise for children and adults alike should be available without being exposed to harmful chemicals.

Of special interest to men, many of whom are golfers, is the use of so many toxic chemicals on golf courses. The U.S. Government Accounting Office (GAO) report of 1990 listed 34 major lawn "care" pesticides, many of which lacked adequate assessments for toxic effects. Six—dichlorvos, (DDVP), maneb, benomyl, pronamide, 2,4-D, and diazinon—were listed as causing one or more of the following: cancer, birth defects, interference with reproduction, mutagenicity, and hazards to wildlife.[47]

Two attorneys general from the state of New York have issued reports on the risk to groundwater from golf course pesticides. Nearly 20% of the pesticides applied to golf courses on Long Island were classified as possible or probable carcinogens, and included propoxur, DDVP, oryzalin, trifluralin, fosetyl-Al, and chlorthalonil. There was one overlap with the GAO and New York state lists; thus, the number of carcinogenic and reproductive products according to those agencies increases to 11. Four common golf courses pesticides identified to cause impairment of nervous function are disulfoton, propoxur, thiram, and chlorpyrifos.[48] A study of 686 deceased members of the Golf Course Superintendents Association of

America, from all 50 states, showed elevated death for four malignancies: brain, non-Hodgkin's lymphoma, intestine, and prostate.[49]

Chlorpyrifos, marketed as Dursban and other names, is one of the most commonly used organophosphate pesticides. I was among a number of experts and victims invited to testify before the U.S. Senate as to the adverse effects from chlorpyrifos exposure. These effects included respiratory dysfunction, neurotoxicity, and birth defects. The testimony from all of the witnesses, as well as my 40-page bibliography, have been made available in the Senate record.[50] Despite compelling information by myself and many others, a Senate bill to simply provide the public with information and notification of pesticide application never became law.[51]

It would be in the best interests of all who participate in sports activities, adults and the parents of children who play sports, to document what chemicals have been used, and to demand chemically free activity areas.

Ordinarily, worldwide, the number of male babies outnumbers females. In Denmark, there has been a change in the male-to-female ratio among newborns,[52] suggesting that this deviation may reflect hormonal and chemical damage, either to the father's sperm or during intrauterine development.[53] Exposure to the agricultural product dibromochloropropane (DBCP) is a suspected agent because it causes depressed sperm counts and a relative increase in female children to be born to exposed fathers.[54] DBCP has been used as a chemical sterilant to combat nematodes and other soil-dwelling species. Widely used in Hawaiian pineapple culture, DBCP has been found in the water supply long after use was discontinued.

Men and women together are suffering from cancer, linked by chemicals, radiation, economics, and politics. When one reads the names of corporate CEOs, their associates, and those on their boards of directors, one realizes that business decisions affecting the health of both men and women are being made primarily by men. Of the top *Fortune-500* corporations, women hold but 643 of a total of 5438 seats.[55] It is unknown if women in business will do a better job of promoting health and safety for all, but given the record to date, it would be worth a try to effect change. Lest I sound anti-male, I note that 1680 scientists, among them 104 Nobel prize recipients, both men and women, signed and published the "World Scientists' Warning to Humanity."[56] Well worth reading, the document stresses that the health of all humanity depends upon stopping the current path of environmental degradation. If not reversed, the ultimate effects will be poverty, social unrest, economic decline, and ultimately, anarchy.

Will it take a major restructuring of business, tax, and legal codes to force business decision-makers to give priority to health and environmental protection above priority for "the bottom line"? Legal, political, economic, and ethical ramifications of corporate behavior are explored in various issues of *Rachel's Environment & Health Weekly,* published by Annapolis-based Environmental Research Foundation. The editor, Dr. Montague, writes: "The environment, democracy, civil society, and the economy are the same problem even though we [mistakenly] consider them separately."[57]

For two-and-a-quarter centuries, in a practically unbroken line, observant citizens and their physicians and scientists have made the connection between various illnesses and exposure to chemicals and ionizing radiation. How much more information is required before prevention is demanded? Can we unite, women and men, to prevent harm to our children and to their children, so that they will not face the needless suffering of cancer, and birth defects, and early death?

REFERENCES

1. Pott, P. Chirurgical Observations relative to the Cataract, the Polypus of the Nose, the Cancer of the Scrotum, the different kinds of Ruptures and Mortification of the Toes and Feet. London. 1775.
2. Hunter, D. The Diseases of Occupations. Little Brown and Co. Boston. p. 819. 1969.
3. Siwek, J. Breast enlargement in boys. Washington Post Health. p. 23. June 24, 1997.
4. Wright, L. Silent sperm. New Yorker. pp. 42–55. January 15, 1996.
5. Bogan, K., County man finds male breast cancer is no joke. Winchester Star. p. B-1. July 18, 1997.
6. Srinivasan, G., Srinivasan, U., Greiver, P. Male breast carcinoma following estrogen therapy: report of a case. J. Ky. Med. Assoc. 77(1): 9–10, 48, 1979
7. World Health Organization. International Agency for Research in Cancer (IARC). Volume 28. 486 pages. 1982.
8. Kreitmair, H., Sieckmann, W. Uber 4,4′-dioxy-diathylstiben, eine synthetische verbindung mit der wirkung des follikelhormons. Klin. Wochenschrift. 156–160, 1939.
9. Hooker, C. W., Pfeiffer, C. A. The morphology and development of testicular tumors in mice of the A strain receiving estrogens. Cancer Res. 2: 759–769, 1942.
10. Cook, J. W., Dodds, E. C., Hewett, C. L. A synthetetic oestrus-exciting compound. Nature. pp. 56–57. January 14, 1933.
11. Cook, J. W., Dodds, E. C. Sex hormones and cancer-producing chemicals.

Nature. 205–206. February 11, 1933.

12. Kipling, M. D., Waterhouse, J. A. H. Cadmium and prostatic cancer. Lancet. 730–731. April 1, 1967.

13. Winkelstein, W., Kantor, S. Prostatic cancer: Relationship to suspended particulate air pollution. Amer. J. Pub. Health. 59(7): 1134–1138, 1969.

14. Chan, J. M. Plasma insulin-like growth factor-1 [IGF-1] and prostate cancer risk: A prospective study. Science. 279: 563–566, 1998.

15. Montague, P. Milk, rBGH and cancer. Rachels's Environment and Health Weekly. #593. April, 9, 1998.

16. Gould, J. M., Mangano, J. J. Prostate cancer mortality rates in nuclear counties. Communique to the International Journal for Health Service. 6 pages. April 14, 1998.

17. Radiation and Health Project, 302 West 86th Street, Suite 11B, New York, NY 10024.

18. Physician's Desk Reference. Medical Economics Co. Inc. Montvale, NJ. p. 1627. 1995.

19. Wright, P. A., Attorney for Dow Chemical Co. Letter to Office of Prevention, Pesticides, and Toxic Substances, U.S. EPA, Re: 3,5,6-trichloro-2-pyridinol. 2 pages. July 24, 1992. (Available under Freedom of Information from U.S. EPA.).

20. Kolata, G. Lack of volunteers thwarts research on prostate cancer. New York Times. p. A-13. February 12, 1997.

21. Sharpe, R. M., Skakkebaek, N. E. Are oestrogens involved in falling sperm counts and disorders of the male reproductive tract? Lancet. 341: 1392–1395, 1993.

22. Carlsen, E., Giwercman, A., Keiding, N., Skakkebaek, N. E. Evidence for decreasing quality of semen during past 50 years. Brit. Med. J. 305: 609–613, 1992.

23. Wilcox, A.J., Baird, D. D., Weinberg, C. R., Hornsby, P. P., Herbst, A. L. Fertility in men exposed prenatally to diethylstilbestrol. New Engl. J. Med. 332: 1411–1416, 1995.

24. Paulozzi, L. J., et al. Hypospadias trends in two U.S. surveillance systems. Pediatrics 11(5): 831–843. 1997.

25. Sherman, J. D. Chlorpyrifos (Dursban)—associated birth defects: A proposed syndrome, report of four cases, and discussion of the toxicology. Internat. J. Occup. Med. Toxicol. 4(4): 417–431, 1995.

26. Sherman, J. D. Chlorpyrifos (Dursban) associated birth defects—Report of four cases. Arch. Environ. Health. 51(1): 5–8, 1996.

27. Sherman, J. D. Dursban revisited: Birth defects, U.S. Environmental Protection Agency, and Centers for Disease Control. Arch. Environ. Health. 52(5): 332–333, 1997.

28. Dow Chemical Co. MSDS, Trichloropyridinol. 3 pages. August 2, 1991.

29. Hanley, T. R., Jr., Zielke, G. J., Lomax, L. G. 3,5,6-Trichloro-2-pyridinol: Oral teratology study in New Zealand white rabbits. Mammalian and Environmental Toxicology Research Laboratory. Health and Environmental

Sciences, Dow Chemical Co., Midland, MI. 148 pages. July 23, 1987. (Available under Freedom of Information from U.S. EPA.)

30. Deacon, M. M., Murray, J. S., Pliny, M. K., Dittenber, D.A., Hanley, T. R., Jr., John, J. A. The effects of orally administered chlorpyrifos on embryonal and fetal development in mice. Toxicology Research Laboratory, Health and Environmental Sciences. Dow Chemical Co., Midland, MI. 109 pages. July 24, 1979. (Available under Freedom of Information, U.S. EPA.)

31. Wright. Op. Cit.

32. Bergstrom, R., Adami, H. O., Mohner, M., Zatonski, W., Storm, H., Ekbom, A., Tretli, S., Teppo, L., Akre, O., Hakulinen, T. Increase in testicular cancer incidence in six European countries a birth cohort phenomenon. J. Nat. Cancer Inst. 88(11): 727–733, 1996.

33. Adami, H. O., Bergstrom, R., Mohner, M., Zatinski, W., Storm, H., Ekbom, A. Testicular cancer in nine countries. Int. J. Cancer. 59: 33–38, 1994.

34. Mills, P. K., Newell, G. R., Johnson, D. E. Testicular cancer associated with employment in agriculture and oil, and natural gas extraction. Lancet. 207–209, January 28, 1984.

35. Ducatman, A. M., Conwill, D. E., Crawl, J. Germ cell tumors of the testicle among aircraft repairmen. J. Urol. 136: 834–836, 1986.

36. Levin, S. M., Baker, D. B., Landrigan, P. J., Monaghan, S. V., Frumin, E., Braithwaite, M., Towne, W. Testicular cancer in leather tanners exposed to dimethylforamide. Lancet. 1153, November 14, 1987.

37. Montague, P. Rachel's Environment and Health Weekly. #547. May 22, 1997. Address: P. O. Box 5036, Annapolis, MD 21403–7036.

38. European Workshop on the Impact of Endocrine Disrupters on Human Health and Wildlife. 2–4 December, 1996. Weybridge. UK Report of Proceedings
(Report EUR 17549) (Copenhagen, Denmark: European Commission DG XII, April 16, 1997.) Available from European Environmental Agency, Kongens,
Nytorv 6, DK-1050, Copenhagen K., Denmark.

39. Colborn, T., Clement, C., Eds. Chemically-Induced Alteration in Sexual and Functional Development: The Wildlife/ Human Connection. Princeton Scientific Publishing Co., Inc. Princeton, NJ. 403 pages. 1992.

40. Bayrische Analine Soda Fabrik chemical company, established in Germany, with worldwide distribution and facilities.

41. Farm Chemical Handbook. Meister Publishing Co. Willoughby, OH. p. C-395. 1995.

42. Kelce, W. R., Wilson, E. M. Environmental antiandrogens: developmental effects, molecular mechanisms, and clinical implications. J. Molec. Med. 75(3): 198–207, 1997.

43. Gray, L. E., Jr., Otsby, J. S., Kelce, W. R. Developmental effects of an environmental antiandrogen: the fungicide vinclozolin alters sex differentiation of the male rat. Toxicol. Appl. Pharmacol. 129(1): 46–52, 1994.

44. Kelce, W. R., Monosson, E., Gamcsik, M. P., Laws. S. C., Gray, L. E., Jr.

Environmental hormone disrupters: evidence that vinclozolin developmental toxicity is mediated by antiandrogenic metabolites. Toxicol. Appl. Pharmacol. 126(2): 276–285, 1994.

45. Yale University Press. New Haven, CT. 380 pages. 1996.

46. Lerda, D., Rizzi, R. Study of reproductive function in persons occupational exposed to 2,4-dichlorophenoxyacetic acid (2,4-D). Mutation Red. 262: 47–50, 1991.

47. U.S. GAO, Lawn Care Pesticides: Risks remain while prohibited safety claims continue. GAO/RCED-90-134. 26 pages. March, 1990.

48. Abrams, Robert, Koppell, G. Oliver. (Separate terms each) Toxic Fairways: Risking Groundwater Contamination From Pesticides on Long Island Golf Courses. New York State, Department of Law. 1994.

49. Kross, B. C., Burmeister, L. F., Ogilvie, L. K., Fuortes, L. J., Fu, C. M. Proportionate mortality study of golf course superintendents. Amer. J. Indust. Med. 29: 501–506, 1996.

50. U.S. Senate, Subcommittee on Toxic Substances, Environmental Oversight, Research and Development of the Committee on Environment and Pubic Works. ISBN 0-16-035481-1. 1991.

51. Senate Bill S.849, 102d Congress. April 18, 1991. Sponsored by Senators Lieberman and Reid.

52. Moller, H. Change in male:female ratio among newborn infants in Denmark. Lancet. 348(9030): 828–829, 1996.

53. James, W. H. Male reproductive hazards and occupation. Lancet. 347: 773, 1996.

54. James, W. H. The human sex ratio, part 1: a review of the literature. Human Biol. 59: 721–752, 1987.

55. Valentine, P. Women in the boardroom: It's not a well-heeled area. Washington Post. p. D-1. November 20, 1997.

56. Full text available from: Union of Concerned Scientists. 2 Brattle Square, Cambridge, MA 02238. Single copies are free, 50 copies cost $3.60.

57. Montague, P., Ed. Rachel's Environment & Health Weekly. #569. October 24, 1997.

14

QUESTIONS, HISTORY, ETHICS, AND MORALITY
THE GLOBAL MARKETPLACE

I think it's time to redefine crime. . . . When corporate executives approve
the dumping of pollution into the air or water, causing untold
environmental damage and eventually killing thousands of people, that
should be a crime. . . . These corporate crimes should be listed as serious
felonies, even more serious than the crimes committed by street criminals.
Why? Because, unlike many of the street criminals who violate the law
because they're high on PCP or are so mentally gone that they can't find an
honest way out of their predicament, the corporate criminal knows exactly
what he is doing and why he is doing it. His motive is pure greed. . . . To me,
that person is a thousand times more criminal and immoral than the crazy
son of a bitch who stole my color TV.
                                         —*Downsize This!* by Michael Moore[1]

Mr. Moore says what needs to be said and says it in a way that leaves no
doubt as to what constitutes crime. While we are assaulted with stories of
"crime in the streets" and treated nightly to the latest TV shooting or high-
profile criminal trial, transnational corporations do as they wish, polluting,
selling dangerous products, not cleaning up their messes, and doing it mostly
hidden from view behind the doors of board rooms, abetted by platoons of
lawyers, public relations firms, paid-for public officials, and dysfunctional
governments.

Why does the United States, admittedly a world leader in wealth, personal comfort, industry, and armaments, have an epidemic of breast cancer? Can it be that the answer lies within the question?

The cancer in our midst is a tragedy, needless, always painful, and inevitably a burden. The burden is to the person with cancer, to her or his family, the community, and to society at large. How much skill, talent, and energy do we lose as each person, one by one, struggles to overcome the silent invader?

The patterns of cancer point clearly to recognizable causes. Major causes involve products and processes, derived from economic and political factors. Remedies are less clear.

If we continue to regulate *chemicals* one at a time, and grant to chemical companies the right to claim their product "innocent" until proven guilty beyond the shadow of a doubt, while ignoring the *process* inherent in the cancer epidemic, we are deceiving ourselves into believing that we will conquer cancer. Nothing could be further form the truth.

The *process* that allows corporations to market chemicals for food production is inherently amiss. Pesticides for crops and drugs for food animals are tested under corporate control and out of the publics' sight. Results of pesticide testing, when submitted to the EPA for "approval" become labeled "business confidentiality" and/or "unpublished." Actually, few people understand that pesticides are not approved by the EPA, but are registered for use. And registered, not based upon EPA testing, but upon corporate testing.

This is inherently the antithesis of a democracy: the right to the free flow of information.

The governmental and the *legal process* allow corporations to promote and market hormones, drugs, and pesticides for crop and food animal use, with little to no oversight or consideration of far-reaching effects. Even the simple measure of labeling dairy products as free from bovine growth hormone (rBGH) was discouraged. Conveniently, the FDA action was written by attorney Michael Taylor, who worked for Monsanto both before and after his tenure as an FDA official.[2] This kind of control gives little recourse to the consumer or farmer who chooses not to use such products.

This is inherently the antithesis of a democracy: the right to the free flow of information, allowing one the right to choose.

Financial interests favorable to the real estate, building, and insurance industries have usurped citizens' rights to choose, to know the hazards, and to achieve recourse when the homes in which they live become contaminated.

State legislatures have passed regulations *requiring* pesticide applications to homes prior to construction and/or sale; have blocked real estate loans when a person decided against such use; and then joined forces to block recourse when the home became unlivable because of the same pesticide contamination.

The citizen's right to avoid chemical exposure has reached the level of the absurd in a little-known Florida regulation. This statute requires that a person who requests to be notified about the application of pesticides on turf before use has to be so designated by a physician certified by the American Board of Medical Specialties in only allergy, toxicology, or occupational medicine.[3,4] This excludes all other physicians, including the patient's own long-term personal physician.

This is inherently the antithesis of a democracy: the right of the person to choose to avoid exposure; the right of a patient to rely on her/his physicians' experience, training, and judgement; and the right of a licensed physician to practice her/his profession within her/his ethical and legal obligations.

But the larger question arises, how did such legislation get written in the first place? Who benefits, and who doesn't?

What has been the consequence of our unfettered economic activities? These activities resulting from decisions carried out far from the communities in which we live? Cancer is one consequence, one with far-reaching ramifications, both as to cause and to result.

We must understand that we cannot contaminate the biosphere; kill off species at our convenience; poison the soil, water, and air with our technologies; and escape the consequences. Nor can we sit idly by while others make decisions to do so.

What right do we have to decide which animal/plant is a pest, and then proceed to kill it? How do we justify the killing off of an entire species, as the dodo and passenger pigeon, hunted to extinction?—the killing of elephants and tigers for trophy parts?—the imperilment of migratory birds by destroying and poisoning their habitat?—the killing of Hawaii's unique birds by pesticides and habitat loss?—the killing of the few wolves, reintroduced into their own native habitat, by ranchers, raising cattle?

What harvest do we now reap, having employed some of the most toxic of poisons in a futile attempt to kill one portion of the animal kingdom, the insects? Insects are still with us, many having mutated to become resistant to our chemical poisons. Insect species were on earth long before we humans made our appearance, and in all likelihood will succeed the human species.

We condone, actively, if not tacitly, the killing of wolves and coyotes in the name of rancher's rights. Do we do this so that we may eat beef grazed on public land, fattened with hormones, and fed on pesticide treated grain? Who was there first, the wolf or the rancher?

We have problems nationwide that require attention, but dominating the news for months were the "OJ" trials, and then the Starr revelations and the Clinton impeachment hearing. Brought out in these trials was the fatal flaw: the need to control. Control has replaced morality, ethics; indeed, control is on its way to overshadow even our concept of God, for now in the name of control, we take away life at will, in the name of business, convenience, and our right to do as we wish.

Such a fatal flaw it is: control.

Cooperation is nearly gone. We now place our children in situations of competition. We teach them that winning is all-important. We encourage "little leagues" instead of providing opportunities for children to cooperate together in a shared activity. We provide public support for competitive sports and cut funds for parks, music, and art. We address crime "prevention" by proposing evening sports. We don't promote learning to *do* something, to *create* something: be it how to make bread, or a table, or a garment; not to *fix* something, be it a car, or a broken faucet; not to *serve* another entity, be it the elderly, children, animals, or our neighborhood.

We tout style, instead of substance . . . always a "new" and "different" mode of clothing, of furniture, of cars. We are bombarded with the messages to want always more, always newer. Can it be that those messages are leading us nowhere?

We pay over $4,000,000 to a single man to play football for 1 year. Can we not pay our teachers commensurately with their efforts and responsibilities? If our children can learn the minutiae of home runs, yards gained, games played, why can't they be taught how their bodies work, how the world's creatures are interconnected, the value of diverse species, the universality of life?

As we become consumers, we cease being creators—we go from active to passive. Thirty years ago, when serving as a physician in a Detroit medical clinic, I was saddened by the passivity of patients who came to the clinic, who simply sat for hours, not reading, not writing, not doing handwork, not doing anything. By definition, clinic patients were low income, but few had any idea as to how to bake bread (15 cents a loaf at that time, one-quarter the price of store-bought bread), few could repair or sew needed garments, few had any idea of how to buy good nutrition on a tight budget. And the city that supported the clinic where I worked didn't seem to notice that unless it taught people skills and provided a sound education, there would never be an end to sick people.

Three decades later, corporate fast food businesses have supplanted meal planning, clothes are not repaired, but discarded, and we celebrate our collective *gross* national consumption.

Today, the "miracle of television" has brought us not universal learning, but children who are passive, with few skills, ever needing to be entertained. And now, even the few "educational" programs, available though Public Television and Public Radio, are under threat of elimination by Congress.

We push our concept of "market economy" on other countries, though they have not the infrastructure to allow citizens to partake. In areas of Eastern Europe and the former USSR, it has had devastating results.

The past 5 years have seen unprecedented mergers and buyouts of already huge corporations—in the name of control. In the medical field, such massing of economic power portends dire consequences. There is control of information so that products can be "targeted" to customers and control of groups of identifiable "health care consumers." That may be read as people with identifiable diseases who offer a potential "market" that can be targeted for "products." There is a massing, in a few hands, of the control of production, distribution, and use of pharmaceutical drugs and appliances; control of the sale and use of medical and laboratory tests; the consolidation and control of hospitals, nursing homes, and home care providers. We are no longer people who become sick. We have become markets. Is it any wonder that prevention receives so little attention? *Cancer is big and successful business!*

There is control by our politicians and governmental agencies in the name of profit. How else can one explain the 25-year hue and cry over the hazards of cigarettes with no definitive action? It was January 12, 1964, when Surgeon General Luther Terry said "the Government would act promptly 'without any foot-dragging,' to decide what can and should be done." He continued: "The Committee considers it more prudent from the public health viewpoint to assume that the established association has causative meaning than to suspend judgement until no uncertainty remains."[5] In other words, he advocated the time-honored public health precept of the *precautionary principle.*

What action was taken by the 1994 Congressional hearings was stopped in its tracks by the tobacco company lawyers until a courageous employee finally blew the whistle, releasing information that had been hidden for years. Despite stonewalling and legal maneuvers; the manipulation of cigarette ingredients; the targeting of sales to children; the insulting specter of seven men, the CEOs of tobacco companies, claiming "cigarettes are not addicting"; the facts finally have become public. These seven tobacco men have yet to be called before a judicial body for lying to Congress and lying to the public. To crown the whole sordid mess, a compliant Congress failed to pass legislation to control tobacco. Public health, public ethics, and public morality fell before the power, money, manipulation, and control of the tobacco industry.

While some protection for United States citizens may emerge from the legislative dance, other countries will get no such protection. In the balance-of-trade arena, the United States exports more than 3 times as many cigarettes as any other country and is the "largest exporter of carcinogens in the world."[6] Witold Zatonski, director of Warsaw's cancer research and treatment center in Poland, complained "you want us to fight for the free world, but how can our children fight for this if your tobacco companies target them as the replacement market for sales Philip Morris and others are losing in the United States?" The message was echoed by the ambassador to Hungary, Mark Palmer, who complained the "United States and it allies worked for 45 years to get the Communists out, and when we did, the Marlboro Man rode into town to claim the victory."[7] As this book goes to press, Congress has yet to address this very profitable product.

Seven Generations is a concept of the Iroquois Nation that embodies living one's life in a way that considers the well-being of the next seven generations. To put the next seven generations in perspective, we must ask ourselves: How many of us know anything about the lives of even four generations of our own family? How our great-grandparents lived, their environment, their health? If we approximate a generation as two decades, four generations go back to 1915. If we add three more generations, or 80 years, it takes us back to 1855. Few know the conditions of life of the mid 1800s. Fewer still can envision what life will be like seven generations hence.

If we do not change our practices, stop polluting, close nuclear power plants, end dependence on agricultural pesticides, provide clean water for humans and nature's plants and animals, what kind of life can the next seven generations look forward to?—An explosion of cancer, birth defects, learning disabilities, poverty, and worst of all, anarchy.

There is no escaping but what has occurred over these years has had a profound impact upon our current health, our current lives, and upon the health and lives of our children and of their children. If life in the future changes as greatly as it has in the recent past, our children and grandchildren are truly in danger. While we have achieved a great many technical advances, many have come at a great price: pollution, sickness, premature death, and environmental degradation. The concept of history, the continuity of the earth, seems on nearly every occasion to have been dismissed. Dismissed, ignored, argued about, challenged, and revised.

We knew about the toxicity of asbestos in 1898, about benzene's hazards in 1862, the predicted carcinogenicity of DES in 1938, and the certainty of DDT's harm in 1952. But we allowed the "experts" to do "one more study," and allowed the interests of business to come before those of the public.

Everywhere environmentalists are under attack. The conscientious, the quiet, the ethical, the hard-working have a tough time to merely exist and do their needed work. To counter the controlling economic and political forces of today is not only difficult, it is nearly impossible.

A few success stories, involving concerted effort and significant economic liability, led to curtailment of the asbestos industry in the United States. The culpability of the industry was abetted by those in the legal profession who used their fine educations to obscure and delay. These dark times of the legal defenders of the asbestos industry have been well documented in Paul Brodeur's *Outrageous Misconduct—The Asbestos Industry Trial*,[8] and Barry Castleman's *Asbestos—Medical and Legal Aspects*.[9] Current legal efforts to overwhelm and subvert the public good are no less adamant. While there was some success in curtailing asbestos exposure in the United States, this was not the case for those overseas, where asbestos manufacturing was transferred to countries lacking worker and environmental protection.

Pesticides, banned in the United States, are manufactured there and sold overseas. After 1987, when chlordane and heptachlor were banned from sale in the United States, the manufacturer continued production in Memphis, Tennessee, from where it was shipped to various United States ports for overseas sale. A clever example of reverse public relations was the May 1997 announcement by Velsicol Chemical Corporation to cease production of chlordane and heptachlor. Contrary to the hoopla that followed the news release about lack of correlation between breast cancer and DDE and PCBs, there was no big announcement in the press, nor by the EPA. The public was simply excluded. Keeping in mind the fact that chlordane/ heptachlor have a half-life of some 40 years, the Velsicol press release bears quoting:

> ...According to Arthur R. Sigel, President and CEO for Velsicol, while chlordane and heptachlor have come to the end of the product life cycle, they have been important products that have saved consumers, farmers and other businesses billions of dollars in damage from termites and fire ants to residential, government and commercial structures, as well as agricultural products. 'We have always believed in the efficacy of these products, and the science that supports their continued use, but the economics no longer support continued manufacture. Our intent is to withdraw from the marketplace in an orderly way, giving our customers sufficient opportunity to complete commitments already made.'

> The orderly withdrawal from the marketplace is a continuation of Velsicol's product stewardship program. Under this program, Velsicol has sold its products to a limited customer base. Uses are approved by each receiving country's regulatory authority and Velsicol.

> ...Velsicol has monitored production volumes of its products as well to ensure it can meet existing obligations to its customers while avoiding the creation of significant inventories after its exit from the business.

> Over the last few years, the products have been used for major road building projects in Africa, protection of residential structures in tropical regions in Northeastern Australia and the Far East, and as a soil insecticide to protect crops in South America.

> ...Velsicol is a privately held specialty chemical manufacturing company headquartered in suburban Chicago [Rosemont], Illinois. The company manufactures products used in plastics, adhesives, coatings, pharmaceuticals, cosmetics and chemical intermediates.

> In addition to its Memphis, TN manufacturing facility, Velsicol has manufacturing operations in Chattanooga, TN, Chestertown, MD, Bayport, TX and Kohila, Estonia, and an environmental consulting and laboratory services business in Memphis.

A week after the Velsicol announcement, Dan Rosenblatt from the EPA Office of Pesticide Programs, International Activities wrote the following to Pep Fuller, also at EPA:

> Subject: Export of the insecticide chlordane. ... As we discussed, there is a fairly onerous clearance process for moving this information to the public domain. Therefore, all years are not yet available. However, we

can work on clearing additional data if you are interested in pursuing this question further.

On the quantity question, for the period 1994 through 1996, Velsicol produced between 3 to 5 million pounds of technical active ingredient for both heptachlor and chlordane. . . . The company also believes that there is another producer in China.

Identifying countries that received shipments, Rosenblatt listed Argentina, Malaysia, Singapore, and India in 1995, and Australia in 1992. What do the owners of Velsicol Chemical Company and the officials at EPA know about the impact on people who have become exposed to these toxic products over the last decade: people both overseas and at United States manufacturing and shipping facilities? International trade is virtually unlimited: can any of us take comfort in the Velsicol and EPA notices?

Disregard for public welfare was implicit in the radiation experiments as well, the full details of which are still not available to the public. Control was and is in the hands of the government and the corporations who ran these facilities, with both chemical and radiation pollution.

The dioxin/PCB/PBB story has not come to conclusion. No definitive methods are in place to prevent, contain, or cleanup these threats to life. Despite overwhelming information to the contrary, some well-supported scientists still claim there is no hazard from exposure.

Undeniably, some technological processes have provided advantages. But far too many have provided only markets, only consumers. A major argument put forth in support of NAFTA was the "creation of markets." Do we the people, the people universal, really need more *things?*

Do we need so many choices? And, are they really choices? Do we need to market everyday products so carelessly and so relentlessly?

Take a critical look at the cereal section of a supermarket. Does anyone need such a variety? Indeed, when one considers that 90% of packaged cereals are made of wheat, corn, oats, and/or rice, sweetened or not sweetened, is there truly a difference? Is this plethora really a choice? How many of us consider the corporate connections when we buy Nabisco cereal products? Do we know that Nabisco is a part of R.J. Reynolds, the tobacco giant?

Do we really think that decreasing the amount of contents of a can or box of product, while keeping the price the same, saves anyone anything? A modest example is the simple can of evaporated milk, relied upon by mothers for generations to ensure a clean and ready supply of milk for their babies. It formerly contained 14 ounces. Now the standard can contains 12 ounces, a 15% reduction, requiring nearly the same amount of metal to make the slightly smaller can. Why have we allowed ourselves to be hoodwinked and our resources squandered? Do we *need* iced tea in a metal can?! How much trouble is it to make a portion of iced tea from scratch?

Do we really want to buy our salad dressings, peanut butters, cooking oils, etc., in *plastic* containers? Someone, somewhere, extracted the crude oil, processed the crude oil into fractions, manufactured the raw plastic, and formulated the plastic containers before they were filled with food. After we use the contents, someone else, somewhere else, will haul them away to an incinerator and/or landfill where they will remain for uncounted time. Do we really want to support such wasteful, polluting, and harmful industries? Do we want to expose others to the toxic components for our own temporary "convenience," and when considering the estrogenic action of some plastics, contribute to our illnesses?

Do we need all the lights on in an office building, day and night? Do we really want to work in sealed-in buildings, without being able to open a window to the morning or evening air? If this excessive reliance upon electricity is connected to oil and coal-burning plants, or to nuclear power plants, can we turn down the power when not needed, and demand power-conserving workplaces?

Do we really want blemish-free fruits and vegetables, cosmetically corrected with dyes and pesticides? Is a weed-free lawn worth the trail of poison extending from the oil fields to the manufacturing plant, to the lawn, to the consumer and his/her family ... and then to the hospital and ultimately the cemetery?

Perhaps the biggest threat from NAFTA and GATT is not the loss of jobs, or the lowering of all of our standards of living, but that we will become a world of *consumers*. Not thinkers, or givers of care and consideration, not silence seekers, not protectors of our world's treasures, not nature appreciators, not helpers of our humankind, but *consumers* of things.

Look about us! What can we change to decrease our reliance upon oil, coal, nuclear power, plastics, chemicals, unneeded services, unwanted products, disposable things? How much of a convenience is polluted water, polluted air, and polluted soil?

Throughout history, nearly every culture has had a moral concept by which it abided, essentially aimed toward preservation of the *common good*, keeping in mind the needs of future generations. Unless *we, each one of us*, become aware of our individual choices, our individual actions, we will not be able to stem the flood of pollution that threatens our very lives. Do we have the ability, the will, to be more than just consumers?

Can we become thinkers? Ponderers? People who can say no, I really don't need that, I really don't want to buy that article it being an unnecessary product of pollution. We understand that individual happiness is derived from good health, a strong family and community, a safe and secure home, peace, and serenity.

Cancer has no place in that scenario.

Can we expect that makers of business decisions will choose the common good over the bottom line?

What is the *common good?* What does the common good for all of the world's people imply, and what does it demand? Can we imagine our world, lived in a righteous manner?

Does it mean the well-being of all the world's citizens? Does it mean protection of resources for the next seven generations? Does it mean that each of us will have to give up some convenience, pay a greater price for something, and do without something to achieve a common good?

What then is the solution?

"Right livelihood," suggest the Buddhists, as was explained by Jean Sadako King, former Lieutenant Governor of Hawaii. In her address before the Fifth International Seminar on Buddhism and Leadership for Peace in Korea, she explained: "Most people would rather earn their living by engaging in work that doesn't harm others or the planet. Greed, of course, mitigates against this and needs to be understood: 1) greed—in terms of the desire not for a reasonable profit but for the maximum possible, regardless of negative impact on human life, animal life, plant life, and the environment; and 2) greed—in terms of the desire for more and more things."[10]

Remember antiwar activists, during the time of Vietnam, who asked, "what if they gave a war and nobody came?" What if we, our families, our children, refuse to pursue our livelihood in needless, toxic industries, producing and using harmful products?

Can we demand of our legislators (local, state, national, and international) levels of responsibility and accountability? Can we demand that the common good be placed ahead of profits, ahead of control?

If women, all of us at risk for breast cancer heed our common good, we *may* be able to exert some effort to achieve the *common good.* Women comprise 50% of the population but not 50% of our legislatures, and women certainly don't occupy 50% of all corporate boards. The only reasonable explanation in the current political climate is that women don't have the financial backing of business interests. It is not too late to make our voices heard.

If those same politicians and corporations, who depend on women as consumers and supporters, don't, won't, or can't protect our next seven generations, then we need to put women and men in charge who can and will. The only way this can be achieved is to enact, monitor, and enforce strong campaign finance laws, and promote a justice system that will ensure justice for all. It is apparent that in many cases, the legal system is not the same as the justice system. As it stands now, the side with the most money, and the cleverest, not necessarily the most ethical, lawyers either wins or delays justice. Never more true is the aphorism "justice delayed is justice denied."

We need to support concerned leaders like Lois Gibbs, who, as a young mother, mobilized efforts to evacuate her neighborhood located adjacent to Love Canal, a dump site filled with toxic chemicals. Ms. Gibbs and her husband, Steve Lester, founded the Center for Health Environment and Justice, then called Citizens Clearinghouse for Hazardous Wastes. Since 1981, the nonprofit organization has provided over 10,000 community-based groups with the tools and skills needed to protect themselves from exposure to toxic chemicals in the environment.[11] Speaking at the 20th Anniversary of the Love Canal crisis, Ms. Gibbs remarked that of the community groups, 80% were led by women. We need to go still further.

Marcia Marks, an activist for health and the environment, reviewed my manuscript and remarked that my writing seems to express anger. She said she was concerned that it might turn off some readers. I value her ideas and thought about them. In reflection, I think my perspective is derived not from anger, but from sadness. In 34 years of practicing medicine, I have seen far too many needlessly injured and sick people to feel complacent about continuing in the same old ways. While medicine offers methods of treatment and a measure of hope and comfort, it provides too little in the way of prevention. Some changes have to be made. When we see, day after day, that our fellow humans are succumbing to the ravages of cancer, I do not understand why we do not raise our collective voices in protest? Do you?

> Ua mau ke ea o ka aina i ka pono—say the Hawaiians—
> The life of the land is perpetuated in righteousness.

REFERENCES

1. Moore, M. *Downsize This!* Crown Publishers, Inc. New York. pp. 110, 111. 1996. Quoted with permission of the publisher.
2. Montague, P. Rachel's Environment and Health Weekly. #593. April 9, 1998.
3. State of Florida. 5E-14.146. Registry of Pesticide Sensitive Persons. Amended 8-11-93.
4. The full story is available on the internet at: http://www.foxbghsuit.com.
5. Washington Post. p. A-1. January 12, 1964.
6. Proctor, R. N. *No time for heroes—Basic cancer research gets all the glory, but known preventive measures could save more lives.* The Sciences. 35(2): 20–24, 1995.
7. Hoagland, J. Joe Camel goes to Europe. Washington Post. p. A-5. April 2, 1998.
8. Brodeur, Paul. *Outrageous Misconduct—The Asbestos Industry on Trial.* Pantheon Books. New York. 374 pages. 1985.
9. Castleman, Barry I. *Asbestos—Medical and Legal Aspects.* Harcourt Brace Jovanovich. New York. 593 pages. 1984.
10. King, J. S. Exploration of right livelihood as one path to peace and justice. Exploration of Ways to Put Buddhist Thought into Social Practice for Peace and Justice. Seoul, Korea. November 18–21, 1991.
11. Center for Health, Environment and Justice. PO Box 6806, Falls Church, VA 22040.
    703-237-2249   e-mail: CCHW@essential.org   web site: essential.org/cchw

15

THE CANCER MOVEMENT
INDEPENDENT, SOLD OUT, OR BOUGHT UP?

Break the Silence—Stop the Epidemic
Open the Doors to Dialogue Around the World

That was the theme of the World Conference on Breast Cancer, held in July 1997, at the University of Kingston, Ontario, Canada. With few trappings, volunteers brought together women from 60 countries, who with virtually a single voice demanded action to stop the carnage.

I learned that the women of Kingston, Canada, like other women living in the Great Lakes Basin, have the second highest breast cancer rate in North America. Why? Kingston shares with other places on the Great Lakes one obvious thing: water. Kingston is a pretty city, situated at the eastern end of Lake Ontario, where the St. Lawrence River begins its journey to the Atlantic. Lake Ontario is last in the chain of the Great Lakes that receive runoff from the states of Minnesota, Wisconsin, Illinois, Indiana, Michigan, Ohio, Pennsylvania, and New York and from the Canadian Province of Ontario. Along the shores of the five Great Lakes are farms, power plants, and industries, adding pesticides, chemicals, incinerator emissions, road runoff, fuels, nuclear wastes, and sewage. There is little wonder that this city, with the multitude of pollutants streaming by, is in the midst of a cancer epidemic.

Needing to stop the epidemic, the women organized. They were led by founder-activist Janet Collins, and Karen Weisbaum, who became president of the organization. Janet Collins describes herself as a "mouthy middle-aged broad." She is outraged by the reluctance of the cancer establishment to speak of the causes cancer and to address prevention in a meaningful way.

The key organizers, 19 women and 1 man, are pictured in The *Kingston-Whig Standard,* the local newspaper that lists the hundreds of volunteers and speakers who made possible the meeting. Against odds, these dedicated people conceived of, organized, and funded an extraordinary meeting.

They understood the pitfalls of relying on corporate sponsorship, in name and practice. Through very hard work, many small fund-raising projects, and keeping the conference modest in setting, the conference was able to foster independence, not beholden to any special interest.

Janet Collins related that during the early stages of organizing the First World Conference on Breast Cancer, they had no money and a telephone bill of some $2000. She turned down an offer of $75,000 from a drug company and a blank check from Dupont.[1] This was at the time when the Canadian Cancer Society estimated that environmental pollution accounted for only about 2% of cancer. The conference accepted major support from Scotiabank and "WeDo" (Women's Environmental and Development Organization), and hundreds of individuals and small independent entities.

WeDo was founded by Bela Abzug, the firebrand former member of the U.S. House of Representatives. Ms. Abzug, a breast cancer survivor herself and not physically well at the time, spoke eloquently of "a Global Nervous Breakdown" and put the crisis in international public health as due to the "malignant development" supporting our lifestyle. Her message was supported by the data on a one-page handout titled "Mother Earth is Sick."

Since one in every eight women will develop breast cancer in her lifetime, and in the entire population, one in three of us will suffer from cancer in one part of our body or another, why is there such complacency?

At the World Conference, international activist Judy Brady, writer and editor of *1 in 3 Women with Cancer Confront an Epidemic*[2] has some ideas. Ms. Brady started out saying that most of us understand why cancer is increasing—"most of us get it . . . cancer is not our fault." She defined the collective cancer establishment: the government agencies of NCI and NIH; the funds-receiving research universities; the ACS, a nongovernmental obedient agency that speaks rarely of carcinogens; and the chemical/pharmaceutical/biotech industry. These businesses, hired and abetted by the public relations industry, are the heart and brain of the cancer establishment.

Since 1971, when President Nixon declared war on cancer, $1,000,000,000,000 have been spent, and there is no improvement in sight. (That's 1 x 10 to the 12th power, a trillion hard-earned dollars!)

Asked why women are not rising up against these issues, Ms. Brady cites economic and job insecurity; unwillingness to take a stand; and the tendency to discount what we know to be true. As for the endless risk assessments under way, she calls them "liars for hire" and wonders how many people it is legal to harm or kill, citing the complicity of "mainstream science as the emperor's tailors." Judy Brady doesn't mince words: we need to listen and understand what she has to say.

One of the high points of the World Conference on Breast Cancer was an address by Sandra Steingraber, a poised and beautiful woman, poet, and holder of a Ph.D. At age 20, Dr. Steingraber learned she had bladder cancer. Since this is uncommon in women, nearly unheard of at that young age, and since she was a nonsmoker and nondrinker, she began to explore why. She learned she was not alone: beluga whales in the St. Lawrence River have been identified with bladder cancer, and they too do not smoke or drink alcohol. And the whales, like the women of Kingston, Ontario, have breast cancer.

"We have a moral imperative to act in the face of inconclusive evidence," says Dr. Sandra Steingraber. Indeed!

Why this concept should be so opposed when it comes to public health is downright immoral. Nearly every other human endeavor is undertaken with incomplete information: bridges span crevasses; starwars weapons are developed; nuclear-containing rockets are shot into space.

Twenty years earlier, Dr. John Gofman said: "I am aware of no instance in the civilian economy where we take it as a premise that injury and murder of members of the public are to be regarded as beneficent acts.[3] Yes, **murder** is the word he used. Think about it! If you or I cause harm, and are told we are causing harm, and don't stop, and it results in death of a person, wouldn't we be put in prison before we could blink an eye? Why have corporations been allowed to escape punishment for the harm they have caused? I mean punishment, not simply pay a fine that is tax deductible, or as it is termed: part of the costs of "doing business."

Self-interest alone dictates that preventing cancer should be the number one priority for all manner of reasons. We hear of thousands convening for the Promise Keepers meeting in 1997, and many more who showed up for the aptly named "Million Man March." And over 97,000 people convened on the second Saturday in October 1997 to watch 22 men who ran, pushed, shoved, and huddled with one another, all for a ball at the Penn State – Ohio State football game. On any one night of a World's Series baseball game, some million people watch in rapt and supportive attention.

What do these events have in common? They are well-organized and well-financed. While the cancer treatment industry is well-organized and well-financed, activists, demanding prevention of cancer, find there is neither. What is lacking in money we do have: dedication. We need strong communication and organization.

Breast cancer advocacy is springing up as a cottage industry. The groups and organizations serve as avenues for support, education, fund raising, and advocacy. Many groups offer needed emotional support to fellow sufferers. Women share their stories, concern about their treatments, their fears. Concerned men receive training in support for their wives. Some groups offer education about treatment options, others offer an opportunity to contribute money and time for the sake of those who are ill and who have few resources for help.

There are several advocacy groups to be applauded: One is the Women's Community Cancer Project, a grassroots volunteer organization, based in Cambridge, Massachusetts.[4] Aware of the environmental causes of cancer and the magnitude of the cancer epidemic, they say: "Women with cancer want the American Cancer Society to confront corporate polluters," rightfully proclaiming "early detection is no prevention." They rightfully emphasize: "Real prevention means not getting breast cancer to begin with."

Another group working on behalf of women is the National Women's Health Network, whose low-cost, easily read publications are straightforward, pointing out the fallacy of "early detection" versus primary prevention. To their credit, members of this network were among those who testified about the hazards of the tamoxifen trials.

However, sometimes these well-meaning groups unwittingly serve the interests of others.

The occasion was the Breast Cancer Awareness Awards luncheon, to honor four outstanding women whose efforts to stem the carnage of this disease deserved accolades. The setting, on a beautiful October day in 1994, was the ANA (All Nippon Airways) Hotel in Washington, D.C. Assembled in the ballroom were 500 well-attired women, all to raise money for the Betty Ford Comprehensive Breast Center at the nearby Columbia Hospital for Women.

First Lady Betty Ford and her contemporary Happy Rockefeller, each with breast cancer, were among the first women to bring into the open the issue of breast cancer. Thanks to them, it became acceptable to talk about breast cancer, to openly discuss mammography, to take away what had been portrayed as shame. Unfortunately, since their coming out, breast cancer incidence has increased 32%.

The artistically designed pink, mauve, and white luncheon program—a statement of refinement and elegance—states with justifiable pride: "Since 1990, nearly 4,000 procedures have been performed, free of charge, for women who would otherwise have had nowhere to turn for the care they needed." This Betty Ford Comprehensive Breast Center is a place where eligible women can receive screening mammograms at no cost, and where, if needed, additional diagnostic mammograms, cyst aspiration, and stereotactic biopsy have been made available. Approximately 167 such procedures were provided to women in 1994. A worthy effort.

The women volunteers had raised $106,000 in 1994, earmarked to provide service for the Low-Income Mammography Program at Columbia Hospital for Women. Barbara Goodman, Co-chair of the Awards Committee, reported the generous contributions of $35,000 from Mobil Corporation, and the program noted contributions from three other benefactors: the Washington, D.C. law firm of Williams and Connolly, the Wyeth-Ayerst Pharmaceutical Corporation, as well as Avon cosmetics.

After the meeting, I called the hospital to find out how one became a "benefactor." A woman told me that one is called benefactor by virtue of giving $5000 or more to the program. Ms. Emerson, the woman who answered my questions, said that gifts traditionally come as a result of friendships between officers of the hospital and vendors. I asked her what she meant by that, but she was reluctant to explain further.

She also said that in the past, Revlon had been a contributor of cosmetic favors for the luncheon, but this year, they were supplied by a different company, Origins. When I asked why cosmetics gifts were a part of the program at all, she replied that the attendees "expect them."

One wonders why any women at the luncheon, who was obviously able to pay her own, at minimum $50, luncheon tab and appeared able to purchase whatever cosmetic, shoes, or clothing she wanted, needs to expect a goodie at all. After all, cosmetic choice is such a personal decision.

Attendees each received a 3 by 4 inch magnetized plastic address reminder for the hospital, suitable for sticking to our refrigerator doors. We were given an

Origins package, containing a half-ounce bottle of "Origins Sensory Therapy—Peace of Mind—On-the Spot Relief." According to the carton, the Origins Commitment, is "Preservation of earth, animal, environment." A worthy goal. Origins other goal is to sell products, and they do so by giving away free samples used to entice customers. It's more than a gift. It's a built-in opportunity to be on the "right" side of the issues and still make a profit. Origins is not alone.

The contents of the bottle, which we were advised to "breath in deeply, massage a tiny dab into neck, temples, forehead, earlobes," were, among many ingredients, the following:

> dimethacone copolyol, poly glyceryl methacrylate, propylene glycol (used in antifreeze), methyl gluceth-20, peg 7 and peg 150, butylene glycol, imidazolidinyl urea, polysorbate 60, tea carbomer 934, dioctyl adipate, methyl, propyl and butyl paraban

Unequivocally, one must applaud the concerned and active women who are trying to stop the carnage of breast cancer and to give support to those suffering with the disease. Understandably, cosmetics may ease the change in our appearance when we are sick, and as we undergo cancer treatment. But, without appearing cranky and mean-spirited, I believe that before ending breast cancer will be a reality, the economic connections must not only be understood, but addressed.

Let's take the last item first. It is apparent that the synthetic chemicals in the Sensory Therapy product are not needed, are possibly harmful, and add to the already overflowing burden of chemicals that surrounds us. In addition, we should even question the little vinyl refrigerator advertisement—a plastic made by the industrial use of chlorine, a chemical that is basic to so much industrial toxicity and a factor in some cancers. Whose mother, sister, daughter was needlessly exposed to these toxic chemicals when she fabricated that unnecessary piece of plastic in some factory? These workers were not the women in attendance at that luncheon. A small note pad of non-chlorine bleached paper with the hospital's address and phone number would have been far more appropriate.

A sponsor, Wyeth-Ayerst, is a major purveyor of estrogens, namely, Premarin. I hope the reader will read, and read carefully, the package insert, and understand that Premarin may be one of the factors adding to our breast cancer load.

As for the law firm listed in the program, Williams and Connolly, their clients include General Electric, a defendant in a number of cases involving damage from carcinogenic PCBs, radiation, and other contaminants. Williams and Connolly waged an all-out campaign to stop the victims in a PCB contaminated area from bringing their claims before a jury. Their attempt was reversed by the Third Circuit Court of Appeals, for the second time, but not before some of the residents died.[5] In the field of breast disease, General Electric, the company that "Brings Good Things to Life," may stand alone in its contribution to a number of illness, including breast cancer. It is, in the words of INFACT, a Boston, Massachusetts, consumer watchdog group, the company that is "spreading a trail of radioactive and toxic contamination ... [and] has created environmental health and safety nightmares across the country."[6] INFACT also reports that "time and time again, GE officials knew that dangerous waste was leaving the Hanford site [home of a nuclear weapons development site] and contaminating people, and that GE clearly understood that the health consequences could be severe. Yet GE never warned the area residents or GE's own workers." And finally, the same report states: "GE ranks number one in Superfund sites, being the 'potentially responsible party' at 51 sites as of August, 1990. [It] also released more cancer-causing chemicals into the environment than any other U.S. company during 1988."[7]

As for the $35,000 benefactor, Mobil Oil, there's a story here too. Mobil, the petrochemical giant, spent hundreds of thousands of dollars fighting its own scientists who warned of harm from its products. In 1990, a jury awarded Mobil employee Valcar Bowman $375,000 in compensatory damages and $1 million in punitive damages after he was fired for refusing to remove documents from the corporations' Bakersfield, California, plastics facility to prevent the documents from falling into the hands of investigators.[8]

In 1994, a jury awarded another Mobil scientist, Dr. Myron Mehlman, $7 million in lost salary and damages after Dr. Mehlman warned of dangerously high levels of the carcinogenic chemical benzene in its Japanese refinery.[9] The Mobil attorneys appealed the jury decision, delaying relief to Dr. Mehlman. On March 26, 1998, the Supreme Court of New Jersey, in an unprecedented ruling, upheld and affirmed the unanimous judgement of the Appellate Division. The opinion written by Supreme Court Justice J. Stein for the majority of the Court says:

> The Conscientious Employee Protection Act . . . a "whistleblower statute" protects an employee from retaliatory action taken against him in New Jersey by his New Jersey employer because the employee objected to a practice that he reasonable believed was incompatible

with clear mandate of public policy to protect the public health and safety of citizens of another Country.

The remainder of the decision also bears repeating:

> There is often very little that prevents industries from introducing toxic and poisonous chemicals and products into the environment. Legislation, written by or in cooperation with industry, cannot be expected to lean toward the best interests of the public and not of the industry. . . . Loyalties to the public and to the employer can be at odds, and the threat of retaliation can be severe and can carry the risk of economic, professional and personal ruin. Very few brave individuals will have the courage to risk their own and their family's well being, comfort, privacy and financial
> security to take the action necessary to protect the public good and prevent potential injury to huge numbers of people. Most find it easier to "look the other way" and not make waves. The New Jersey Supreme Court ruling in Mehlman v. Mobil Oil should encourage and provide the protection necessary for courageous individuals to speak out when chemical, pharmaceutical, petrochemical and oil companies, nuclear facilities, waste disposal companies and others act or plan to act in a manner that poses serious danger to the public and the environment.

Mobil not only contributes to breast cancer groups, but it is the same company that "gives money to the Heritage Foundation, a right-wing think tank that has proposed opening designated federal wilderness to strip mining. Heritage has called upon conservative activists to 'strangle the environmental movement' and thereby put an end to 'the greatest single threat to the American economy. . . .' Mobil [also] helps fund Citizens for the Environment, a Washington-based lobbying group that believes environmental problems would be solved if only corporations were deregulated."[11]

So much for sponsors and underwriters. Their financial support may be welcomed, but they have more than one side, and it is well to know with whom you ally yourself.

But back to the October luncheon. Looking at the women who attended the event, one must conclude that most are financially able, educated, and well-meaning. What is missing is knowledge of the issues; else why would one accept, without question, such a setup as that luncheon? When I tried to raise the issue of the causes of breast cancer with one of the physicians in attendance, I received only a polite nod. I tried on a one-to-one basis to stir up a conversation with several women wearing the identifying pink ribbon. I was successful with only one woman, Judy Ochs, who it turns out is a driving force in the Pennsylvania Breast Cancer Coalition. Judy told me she first found she had breast cancer when she was but 46 years old, and then, because of a series of medical mishaps, requested a second mastectomy. She had cancer in her remaining breast. Exceedingly bright, Judy has a sparkle, a sense of humor, and a sense of outrage about the breast cancer epidemic in her area. She told me that Pennsylvania has the fourth highest breast cancer rate in the nation. (New York, California, and Florida vie for top honors). Pennsylvania also has Three Mile Island nuclear plant, and the largest number of Superfund sites in the nation. Judy is particularly concerned about the number of women diagnosed with inflammatory breast cancer in the Lancaster area. Because inflammatory breast cancer is relatively uncommon and may be a marker for specific exposures, Judy has tried many avenues, without success, to get help to assess the women and their environment.

Shortly after our meeting, Judy invited me to Lancaster to speak on toxic chemicals and their connection to cancer. Later I spoke at the Pennsylvania Breast Cancer Coalition meeting in Harrisburg. As Judy and I were taking the elevator after the meeting, a friend of hers approached and said "Oh, you must be Dr. Sherman. Judy told me about you, but I decided not to come to your talk because I was afraid of what you would have to say." Judy is not afraid to hear about chemicals, radiation, and cancer: in fact, with her keen sense of reality and enthusiastic personality, she is a leading patient advocate for primary prevention. Understandably, after surgery and chemotherapy, Judy said she did not want to undergo any more procedures. But, over the next 5 years, doing her own extensive research online and in medical libraries, she determined she did want to have breast reconstruction; she determined what type to have; and who was the most likely surgeon to do it. My husband and I visited her in the hospital 2 days after her surgery, and the first thing she did was pull up her gown, and say "look at these fine hooters!" Judy is not simply a survivor, she is a thriver!

At the Breast Cancer Awareness awards luncheon, conversations were restrained, polite, and controlled. Real issues, involving pollution, carcinogens, and prevention were avoided and, for those who are knowledgeable about the issues, the message of the luncheon was frustrating, despite the pleasure of honoring Dr. Devra Lee Davis for her significant contributions to awareness of cancer causation.

A prime example of corporate control is the annual October Breast Cancer Awareness Month (BCAM). According to "BCAM SCAM," an exposé published in *The Nation,* the BCAM idea "was conceived and paid for by a British chemical company that both profits from this epidemic and may be contributing to its cause. Imperial Chemical Industries (ICI), along with two nonprofit groups, cofounded BCAM 9 years ago. The October event has grown in influence, with 13 institutions now on its board, which includes the American Cancer Society and the National Cancer Institute. BCAM has become fashionable too: Avon, Estée Lauder, and Hanes have lent sponsorship. But, since the beginning, all BCAM's bills have been paid by Zeneca Pharmaceuticals, the new name of ICI's United States subsidiary. Altogether, ICI has spent several million dollars on BCAM, according to [a] Zeneca spokeswoman."[12] For this support, ICI can control the message: "Early detection is your best protection."

Janet Collins thinks the better message is "Prevention is your best protection." We have no trouble accepting immunization for our children and thus have decreased suffering and death from polio, whooping cough, tetanus, diphtheria, and the like. Why do we accept less than true prevention when it comes to cancer? Janet also says: "This practice of polluting corporations recruiting women as their spokespeople drives me crazy. Not only do they get to give the impression that they are equal opportunity and that women are with them side-by-side in the march of progress, but the cowards get to hide behind the skirts of women."[13]

Early detection is important, because like other cancers, breast cancer is more curable before it has spread. But, detection is not prevention: ICI is in the business of manufacturing and selling synthetic chemicals. With annual sales well in excess of $18 billion, ICI is one of the world's largest producers and users of chlorine.

And, as discussed earlier, ICI/Zeneca manufactures tamoxifen (brand name is NOLVADEX), the world's top-selling cancer drug used for breast cancer. Breast cancer activists must understand that what is good for a corporate sponsor may not be in the interest of the activist.

I attended the May 1994 National Breast Cancer Coalition (NBCC) meeting, billed as "Practical skills for political solutions." Speaker Tom Sheridan said: "Democracy is not a spectator sport—ask for accountability," and Congresswoman Marjorie Margoles Mezvinsky reminded us that after 451 years and a total of 3777 different members of Congress, only 163 had been women. The solution to stopping cancer lies in the political and economic area, not the medical. We already have more than enough information to take action.

The NBCC conference packet included a handout that under Prevention, stated: "Etiology: Must know the cause—not clear at this time." Listed under moderate risk were "upper socioeconomic status" and "significant radiation to the chest." Not defined was "significant" and completely absent was the issue of the more significant source of radiation, that of radioisotope contamination of ourselves and our food supply. Under "questionable" risks NBCC listed oral contraceptives and hormonal replacement therapy. Don't these leaders get it? Judy Brady got it, why don't they?

Can this lack of attention to toxic chemicals and nuclear radiation as factors in causation of cancer be in any way connected to the sponsors listed on the program? These corporations are in the business of marketing chemical products: cosmetics, solvents, plastics, pesticides, surfactants, and pharmaceuticals. Can activists expect that such companies will continue to back us if we advocate cutbacks in the use of chemicals if cutbacks reduce sales?

Clearly, accepting gifts and underwriting funds poses problems for the independence of the environmental groups. There was concern that because of pressure, and the difficulty of raising funds, the Kingston group who sponsored the First World Conference on Breast Cancer may not emphasize prevention when they next meet in the year 1999. Self-preservation alone demands a strong stance, but as they well know, not accepting gifts and underwriting poses problems as well, mostly the starvation of advocacy work. This year, Greenpeace closed offices and curtailed operations because of lack of money. Sierra Club is in a similar situation, as is Environmental Health Network, the organization that researched and published *Inconclusive By Design*.

While advocacy groups are cutting back because of lack of funds, financial support for groups such as the Center for Risk Analysis and the Health Policy and Management Department, based at the Harvard School of Public Health, is thriving. A partial list of donors includes the following:[14,15]

Aetna Life and Casualty Co.

ARCO Chemical Co.

Alcoa Foundation

American Automobile
   Manufacturers Assoc.

American Crop Protection Assoc.

American Petroleum Institute

Ashland Oil, Inc.

Astra USA, Inc.

Atlantic Richfield, Co.

BASF Corp.

Bethlehem Steel Corp.

Chemical Manufacturers Assoc.

Chevron Corp.

CIBA-GEIGY Corp.

Citco Petroleum Corp.

Coca-Cola Co.

Cytec Industries, Inc.

Dow Chemical Co.
DowElanco (now DowAgro)
Edison Electric
E. I. DuPont de Nemours & Co.
Eastman Chemical Co.
Electric Power Research Inst.
Exxon Corp.
Ford Motor Co. Fund
Frito-Lay, Inc.
General Electric Foundation
General Motors Corp.
Georgia-Pacific Corp.
Glaxo Wellcome
Goodyear Tire and Rubber Co.
Grocery Manufacturers of
    America
Hoechst Celanese Corp.
Hoechst Marion Roussel
Hoffman-LaRoche, Inc.
ICI Americas, Inc.
International Paper
Janssen Pharmaceutica, Inc.
Johnson & Johnson
Kansas Health Trust

Kraft General Foods, Inc.
Marion Merrill Dow, Inc.
Mead Corp.
Merck & Co.
Minnesota Mining &
    Manufacturing Co.
Mobil Foundation, Inc.
Monsanto Co.
National Steel
New England Electric System
Olin Corp.
Oxygenated Fuels Assoc., Inc.
PepsiCo, Inc.
Procter & Gamble Co.
Reynolds Metals Co., Foundation
Rhone-Poulenc, Inc.
Rohm and Haas Co.
Shell Oil Company Foundation
Texaco, Inc.
Union Carbide Corp.
Unocal
Upjohn Co.
Westinghouse Electric Co.
WMX Technologies, Inc.

It is not illegal for a corporation to fund studies that are in its financial interest. It is folly to underestimate such financial power, and imperative to document and understand that kind of power. When Harvard University (and other similarly funded groups) releases policy and risk statements on environmental and health issues, we must heed the advice: **follow the money!**

Breast Cancer Action (BCA) did.[16] This advocacy group, based in San Francisco, stated: "Under no circumstances will policy or program decision be affected by the people or companies who donate support to the work of Breast Cancer Action. We cannot be bought, influenced or discouraged in our mission to eradicate breast cancer." As one of its guiding principles, "BCA advocates the precautionary principle of public health that calls for acting on the weight of evidence that links environmental carcinogens to breast cancer and other cancers, rather than waiting for absolute proof of cause and effect. Consistent with position, Breast Cancer Action will not knowingly accept funding from corporate entities whose products of manufacturing processes directly endanger environmental and/or occupational health or may possibly contribute to cancer incidence, nor will Breast Cancer Action knowingly accept donations from corporate entities that work to weaken or circumvent environmental or occupational regulations that would protect the public health."

Contrasted to the list of donors acceptable to the Harvard Center for Risk Analysis, Breast Cancer Action made the policy decision not to accept contributions from the following categories:

1. Pharmaceutical companies
2. Chemical manufacturers
3. Oil companies
4. Tobacco companies
5. Health insurance organizations
6. Cancer treatment facilities

We certainly live in a unique time. Just a few years ago, one would have thought that advocates on behalf of health and prevention of cancer could embrace the support of pharmaceutical companies and cancer treatment facilities. Reflecting on the purpose of the corporation to sell products and services and maximize profits, it becomes apparent that prevention cannot be in the interest of the bottom line. What a sad and bitter realization.

The breast cancer issue has been adopted not only by pharmaceutical corporations, but by advertising for fashionable products and meetings. All the while, laws protecting polluters remain in place and the polluters co-opt advocacy groups. We must understand the false allure of the powerful and rich, of luncheon perks, and products that add to our contaminated lives. We must understand the sources of authority in our culture, end naivete, take charge of our own lives, and raise our own funds by dint of our own labor. Can we, as Breast Cancer Action did, learn to say, "No thank you" to tainted money? Even a small amount of tainted money? The $35,000 gift to the Breast Cancer Awareness luncheon donated by Mobil may sound like a lot, but it is less than one-half of 1% of only two jury judgements against Mobil. And that total does not count the money spent on attorneys, fighting citizen's concerns, and opposing concerned and honest scientists.

A look into the gift horse's mouth may reveal rotted teeth and very bad breath.

REFERENCES

1. Collins, Janet. Personal communication. April 14, 1998.

2. Brady, Judith, Ed. 1 in 3: Women with Cancer confront an Epidemic. Cleis Press, Pittsburgh, PA. 286 pages. 1991.

3. Gofman, J. W. An Irreverent Illustrated View of Nuclear Power. Committee for Nuclear Responsibility, Main POB 11297, San Francisco, CA 94101. p. 140. 1979.

4. Women's Cancer Center, 46 Pleasant Street, Cambridge, MA. 02139. Telephone: 617-354-9888.

5. U.S. Court of Appeals for the Third Circuit. Re: Paoli railroad yard PCB litigation. No. 92-1995. August 31, 1994.

6. "Bringing Good Things to Light." A booklet, researched and compiled by INFACT, Boston, MA. October 1990.

7. "Bringing GE to Light." A report, researched and compiled by INFACT, Boston, MA, October, 1990.

8. Hamilton, M. M. Fired Mobil employee wins $1.375 million judgement. Washington Post. p. B-18. November 22, 1990.

9. Anon. Fired Mobil scientist awarded $7 million. Science. 264: 656, 1994.

10. Dr. Myron A. Mehlman v. Mobil Oil Corporation, et al. (A-5-97), decided, New Jersey Supreme Court, March 26, 1998.

11. Bleifuss, Joel. "Rights, Responsibilities and the Press." In These Times. November 29, 1993. pp. 12–13.

12. Paules, M. BCAM Scam. The Nation. p. 558. November 15, 1993.

13. Collins, Janet. Personal communication. April 1998.

14. Harvard Center for Risk Analysis. Harvard School of Public Health. A Joint Annual Report. 20 pages. 1995.

15. Crowley, E. Follow the Money. Breast Cancer Action. 55 New Montgomery, Suite 624, San Francisco, CA 94105. p. 5. October/November 1997.

16. Breast Cancer Action. 55 New Montgomery, Suite 323, San Francisco, CA 94105. 415-243-9301. www.bcaction.org

16

WHAT THE CITIZEN CAN DO

PERSONAL CHOICES AND POLITICAL ACTIONS

To be the eyes and ears and conscience of the Creator of the Universe. . . .
—Kurt Vonnegut[1]

That was fictional Kilgore Trout's answer to the question "what is the purpose of life?" If we are not the conscience of the Creator of the Universe who shall be? If we keep this concept in mind, perhaps our collective actions can reverse the scourge called cancer. Reversing the cancer epidemic will require effort, both personal and public. Personal effort to become educated as to the facts and the issues to protect our own lives and those of our family, and public effort to change the dangerous course on which we find ourselves, locally, nationally, and internationally.

On a personal basis, much information given to patients is insufficient to make informed choices, and much information is incorrect. Not everyone has the will, the resources, the energy, or the guts to do extensive medical research in cancer causes and treatment options, but the least we must do is to ask questions, demand answers, and consider options.

Judy Ochs, the breast cancer survivor/thriver and advocate for care and prevention, the woman described in the previous chapter, is a prime example. This is her story, in her own words, with some names and places omitted to protect the "innocent/guilty":

> This is how my journey began. I was having routine mammograms done every two years after age 40. (I had a benign lump removed from

my breast in '79.) I had a tubal ligation done a short time after my second marriage in '86 and for the first time, my periods became very irregular and my premenstrual symptoms much more pronounced. I had lots of breast tenderness with radiation down both arms, the right always worse than the left. I could feel an area of thickening in my right breast, but no lump. So I was not surprised when they asked to do additional films on my right breast in August of '91. (I was 46.) An ultrasound was also done that day on a lesion that was visible on my mammogram and a biopsy was suggested. I networked my way through the medical system and got the name of the #1 "breast" surgeon here in AAAA—a female. I thought I was in excellent hands, and even had one of the physicians where I worked make a personal contact. I had my biopsy done under local anesthesia so I was very much awake when she entered the OR and a nurse said to her, "Judy's films are here. Do you want them up?" And she replied tersely: "No, I know where I'm going!" (sigh.) If I knew then what I know now, I would have opened my mouth. Unfortunately, I did not. Consequently, my lump was missed and the surgeon instead removed the area of thickening. Local pathology struggled with the diagnosis saying it appeared to be severe atypia, but because they were uncertain they sent the slides to a doctor at the University of BBBB who had written a book on breast pathology, and who pronounced it LCIS [Lobular Carcinoma in situ]. Slides were also sent to the University of CCCC and to DDDD Medical Center. Both came back as severe atypia. I was in cancer kindergarten at that point. But something inside me kept telling me I was in trouble and that I needed to keep myself moving to save my life. In October I self-referred myself to Dr. EEEE at the University of CCCC. I was told he was one of the top four surgical oncologists in the nation. I waited nearly three hours to see him, had to help a foreign medical student take my history, had to recover my films which were somehow switched with another patient's, and then endured his cursory exam which lasted all of five minutes. He examined my breasts and ignored my concern over what felt like a lump to me in my right breast. He backed out of the room saying "I agree with your surgeon from AAAA, and by the way, I'm doing a study on Tamoxifen and if you would like to be a part of it call me in January 1992." I returned to my surgeon in January '92 for a repeat mammogram. That day remains frozen in time. The technician came in the room and said "your lump is still there and it's bigger." That was my turning point. That was the day I realized that in order to get good medical care I had to be an active participant in my care. I responded "those are my films and this is my body; bring me the films; I want to see them." I did see them and was devastated. However, I was also educated by this time and knew immediately that I needed to have a needle localization in that breast and that I wanted to have a biopsy done on my left breast because of the diagnosis of LCIS and the high likelihood of its mirror image occurrence. I returned to the original surgeon who did as I requested. I was diagnosed with infiltrating ductal carcinoma in my right breast and was told the left was negative. By this time a number of negative events had occurred and I started to again network through the medical community, asking where to go. I heard the name Hopkins [Medical Center] over and over. I had a professional friend make a phone call and he found Dr. FFFF, a medical oncologist for me. Three days after my biopsies I was sitting with her as she reviewed my medical reports, the slides, and path reports. I told her I wanted to have bilateral mastectomies. She matched me with Dr. GGGG, a surgical oncologist. He asked me what I wanted of him and I told him that unless he advised me otherwise, I wanted a modified radical [mastectomy] on the right and a simple on the left. He explained that to do the simple on the left would be considered to be prophylactic—I told him I didn't care what he called it, I just wanted it done. He complied with my wishes and my final pathology report on my left breast showed an area of LCIS!! I was home in 48 hours after my surgery (by my choice). I had two nodes positive and underwent six cycles of CAF (cytoxin, adriamycin, and fluorouracil). Surgery was February '92—I was 47.

Ms. Ochs' account bears study. Not everyone experiences inattentive and distracted physicians, but many do. If we are to save our own lives we must speak up and insist on answers and clarification when there is *any* chance of misunderstanding. We cannot foresee the future, but we can make certain assumptions based upon past experience, and it is reasonable to say that if Ms. Ochs had not taken her medical care into her own hands, we would not have this powerful advocate with us today.

There are other messages within her account. Atypical cells are not normal cells, else they would not be called *atypical.* This diagnosis requires close attention and follow-up. Atypical cells represent a change in the scheme from normal to dysplasia and metaplasia, to frank malignancy. With roots in Latin, *in situ* means cells in their "original situation." These are cells that give the appearance in a pathology specimen to have not (yet) spread. Carcinoma *in situ* is a true malignancy, with all the features of malignancy.

In situ bears mentioning again. Recalling the Long Island Breast Cancer Study, none of the women with cancer *in situ* were in the group chosen to have assays of their blood or urine. Appreciating that these women were diagnosed with malignancy, but before their cancers had spread, it is more than unfortunate that assays will not be done for these women. Their unique findings may help define what conditions exist during the transition from normal, to *in situ* (contained) cancer, to cancer that has spread.

Dr. EEEE offered to Ms. Ochs participation in a tamoxifen trial. We do not know the effects of tamoxifen on women with atypical breast cells, nor on women with carcinoma *in situ*. We do know that women with a prior biopsy showing atypical ductal hyperplasia or atypical lobular hyperplasia have increased risk of being diagnosed with breast cancer. Pre-menopausal women with the atypical lobular abnormality have an even greater risk.[2]

Curiously, the NCI Press Office release of April 6, 1998, in discussing what factors were used to determine who was eligible to participate in the tamoxifen prevention trial, said: "Women diagnosed as having lobular carcinoma *in situ*, a condition that is *not* (emphasis added) cancer, but indicates an increased chance of developing invasive breast cancer, were eligible on that diagnosis alone."[3] Also included were women with atypical hyperplasia. What the NCI press release fails to tell us is the outcome of the women who began participation, having abnormal, cancerous cells. Did tamoxifen prevent a progression from *in situ* to invasive cancer for those women? Did follow-up biopsies show the same lesion, a return to normal, or spread of their malignancy? Were any of the women, having what many pathologists diagnose as malignant lesions[4] lulled into complacency by being a part of the "prevention" trial? And on what basis does the NCI categorize lobular carcinoma *in situ* as not cancer, when data shows that it progresses to invasive cancer more frequently than ductal carcinoma *in situ* (DCIS)?

A powerful lesson in the consequences of being active or passive comes with Ms. Ochs' account. Active participation is a requirement for good medical care, whether it is to treat diabetes, liver disease, or cancer, and our active participation may make the difference between life and death. So too, must we be active, cease being passive and take steps to prevent cancer.

On a national basis we learn of pesticides in our foods and are urged to buy organic foods and drink purified water. But this is not enough, for what is to save the less-well-off, the poorly educated, or the family, unaware of hazards? Unless the common good is provided, none will be safe. The benefits of widely available public health programs has been proved again and again by such publicly funded programs as immunizations, water and sewage treatment, and public education. Health and safety must not be the province of only the well-educated and the well-off. **Every** family should be able to obtain water, food, and air, free from chemical and radiological contamination. In the long run, what is more humane and cost-effective than to **prevent** cancer?

We must demand an end to drug- and pesticide-tainted foods. We must demand the closing of nuclear power plants. And we must pursue a paradigm shift in how we deal with waste. If dump sites are filling and causing pollution, and incinerators are spewing toxic wastes over the land and waters, we must institute comprehensive plans to reduce waste at the onset. One step at a time, we can each use less power, take care not to create waste, support local organic agriculture, and eat "lower on the food chain." This means consuming legumes and grains for our source of protein.

There will never be a time when we know every aspect of breast cancer, how it evolves, and its many causes. We do know from studies of worldwide populations that breast cancer, as with every other cancer, is not randomly distributed in any population, not at any time in history, and not anywhere in the world.[5] And breast cancer is increasing, especially in industrialized countries.[6] Is this what we should accept as "progress"? Progress toward what?

For instance, we know that women living in some areas develop breast cancer more often than women in other areas. When women from Japan move to the United States, their breast cancer incidence increases. This difference is accounted for by the environment. In this context, environment includes where and how we live and work, and the total content and sources of our air, food, and water. We understand that early diagnosis may be useful, but it is not prevention. We understand too that continuing the status quo, remaining passive and not acting on the information we already have, however incomplete, will doom still more women to the physical and mental assaults of breast cancer. It is for these reasons we must take collective action to stop the current random killing. Random murder, Dr. John Gofman calls it.

The summer of 1997 brought good and bad news for cancer victims: victims present, past, and future.

August 1997 carried the news that thousands are at risk to develop thyroid cancer as a result of radioactive iodine, drifting from the inactive, but still contaminated, Nevada nuclear test site. The director of NCI, Richard Klausner, announced that between 10,000 and 75,000 Americans may develop thyroid cancer.[7] Additional plausible cancers, not mentioned, were those to result from exposure to radioactive cesium, strontium, carbon, and other elements released in the explosions. Surprise!

Quite by coincidence that same day, I read the slim volume of Congressional hearings titled "Fallout from Nuclear Weapons Tests."[8] That particular hearing was held in 1959. Sitting on that committee were Albert Gore from Tennessee and Henry Jackson from the state of Washington. It was the former, whose son became the current U.S. Vice-President, and the latter, whose state became home to the Hanford nuclear facility, perhaps one of the most contaminated places on earth this side of Chelyabinsk and Chernobyl. The book reported, that by 1958, with aboveground nuclear tests, as much as 40 microcuries of radioactive strontium (Sr 90) per square mile of land had fallen in the northern latitudes, and predicted the level to reach 80 microcuries by 1965.[9] Discussed and predicted also in the book were adverse effects to *present and future generations, now ignored and forgot.*

While the radiation issue was a portion of the bad news, the good news occurred at the SecondWorld Conference on Breast Cancer in the summer of 1999. The conference, organized by outraged women from Kingston, Ontario, Canada, together with supporters from other organizations (WEDO, Greenpeace, and the Women's Network on Health and Environment) brought together 1600 delegates from some 60 countries. The good news was not that the breast cancer rate has decreased in the United States and Canada, or that it is not increasing in other countries. The good news was the message that we the delegates have had enough of "studying the problem," coming up with inconclusive results, and doing nothing about prevention.

A myriad of scientific papers exist concerning adverse effects from exposure to radiation and from exposure to hundreds of chemicals. There is more than enough information to make informed decisions about exposure to these entities. We must insist on the *precautionary prinicple*, that is, to take action to prevent illness, in the face of incomplete data.

Why is prevention not instituted when a product or facility is known to carry harm? Is it that some commercial venture will "lose" money if a product is curtailed?

A more sinister question is the part played by the business of medicine and its allies. These include the chemical and pharmaceutical manufacturing industry—often the same entity; the United States' misnamed private "health care" industry with its seven-figure CEOs; and the uncounted number of medical facilities and their personnel, built to look after the sick and dying, who do little to nothing to prevent illness.

Logically, if the cost of "health care" is threatening to bankrupt an economy, shouldn't that argument drive prevention? Unfortunately, the day has arrived when people openly argue that we can't prevent harm to some portion of our population because it will put someone out of a job and cost a business its profit. This argument has been rendered transparent as tobacco companies urge owners of stores, restaurants, and sports facilities to join in opposing restrictions on cigarettes, as if they were someway protected from cancer. Less transparent are the arguments, pitting jobs versus the environment, but labor action—such as that fought by Caesar Chavez on behalf of farm workers—has demonstrated you can have more and better jobs in healthier and safer workplaces. Given that the United States alone of major countries does not have universal single-payer medical care, it appears that the "health care" industry is thriving, and it is unlikely that either it or the allied industries benefiting from the sick are going to lead the charge for prevention.

Who then will demand prevention?

The same people who have always led the charge. Those who led the fight to end slavery; to obtain civil rights for all; to obtain voting for all citizens; to stop the building of nuclear power facilities and toxic incinerators; to stop the war in Vietnam. The same people who are outraged by the status quo of waste, sickness, needless early death, loss of human potential, and loss and degradation of the world's resources.

If our governments, the elected and civil servants, the transnational businesses, and the "health care" industry are not willing or able to achieve prevention, then we the citizens can and must. We can and must educate ourselves and the public at large about the known hazards from radioactive and chemical pollution. We cannot outspend nor out-PR the polluting opposition, but we can, one by one, each of us, act and vote at the polls and vote with our pocketbooks. We can starve the opposition when we find their actions and products unacceptable. We can refuse to buy the products from corporations that pollute and harm. We can raise our voices, singly and as a chorus of outraged citizens, and make nonstop protestations against immoral polluting activities. We can support groups fighting for a cleaner, safer, saner planet. For those, weary and sick, we can give our support to those younger and stronger who carry on the battle. And battle it is, for our lives and for the lives and well-being of our children and grandchildren. For many it is too late to prevent cancer, but it is not too late to take action to prevent cancer in our children and grandchildren We are the keepers of our sisters, brothers, and children. If not we, then who will keep them safe?

Pray for the dead, and fight like hell for the living!

—Mother Jones, Labor and Human Rights Organizer (1830–1930)

REFERENCES

1. Vonnegut, Kurt, Jr. Breakfast of Champions. Dell Publishing Co., Inc. New York. p. 67. 1973.

2. Marshall, L. M., Hunter, D. J., Connolly, J. L., Schnitt, S. J., Byrne, C., London, S. J., Colditz, G. A. Risk of breast cancer associated with atypical hyperplasia of lobular and ductal types. Cancer Epidemiol. Biomarkers and Prevention. 6: 297–301, 1997.

3. NCI Press Office. Questions and Answers: The Breast Cancer Prevention Trial. 12 pages. April 6, 1998.

4. Chandrasoma, P., Taylor, C. R. Concise pathology. 2nd edition. Appleton and Lange. Norwalk, CT. p. 252. 1995.

5. Segi, M. Graphic Presentation of Cancer Incidence by Site and by Area and Population—Cancer Incidence in Five Continents. Segi Institute of Cancer Epidemiology. Yomeicho 2–5, Mizuho-ku, Nagoya, 467, Japan. 1977.

6. Davis, D. L., Hoel, D. Trends in Cancer Mortality in Industrial Countries. Annals N. Y. Acad. Sci. 609: 1–345, 1990.

7. Suplee, C. Thyroid cancer may threaten thousands exposed to nuclear fallout, study finds. Washington Post. p. A-3. August 2, 1997.

8. United States Congress. Fallout from Nuclear Weapons Tests. Joint Committee on Atomic Energy. 86th Congress. U.S. Government Printing Office. Washington, D.C. 42 pages. 1959.

9. Marshall et al. Op. cit.

17

SOURCES OF INFORMATION AND ACTION
KNOWLEDGE IS POWER

Libraries are full of information about the part played by toxic chemicals and ionizing radiation in causing not only breast cancer, but the many other cancers that are killing men, women, and children. These concepts are not a novel and the information is not particularly new. Today, indeed for decades, **there exists enough information about nearly every chemical used in commerce, the home, and agriculture to determine its potential for risk.** We do not need to reinvert the wheel! **Well-established as well is scientific information concerning hazards of ionizing radiation. We must use the information to take preventive action.**

LITERATURE SOURCES

Regulatory statutes and data are available from state, federal, and provincial governmental sources. In the United States, information is available from governmental agencies: EPA, OSHA, NRC/AEC/DOD, CPSC, NIOSH, FED, NIEHS, NCI, and so forth. In Canada, England, and elsewhere, information is available from comparable governmental sources.

With the rapid development of internet access and computer data bases, information is available online for no cost or for very low cost. The U.S. National Library of Medicine, based in Bethesda, Maryland, maintains the Grateful Med and other computer data bases, allowing any person to find information on diseases, drugs, treatments, toxicology, radiation, mammography, carcinogens, radiation, etc., etc.

Despite the convenience of online data bases, the time-honored practice of going to the library is strongly encouraged. It is there, in the actual medical journals that you will find not only scientific publications but the trail of evidence: the advertising for drugs and procedures, many now implicated in the epidemic of illness. In the agricultural journals you can find advertising for animal growth-promoting drugs and pesticides that are now implicated in so many adverse effects upon humans and the environment. The business and commerce sections of libraries contain fascinating information on questionable technology. Advertising supporters and editorial boards of various publications give insight into potential for bias.

For the person addicted to libraries, and I am one, it is the older publications, not yet available on computer data bases, where you will find the early literature linking disease to various chemicals or ionizing radiation. The time-honored process of obtaining each article on a bibliographic "tree" and going back in time to the first article on a subject is interesting, and it is where you will find who knew what and when they knew it. By this process we often discover that information on a subject has been known for decades. While more recent or more sophisticated scientific studies may become available, the earlier reports serve as valuable warnings.

The following citations are intended to give the reader food for thought, an expanded point of view, and provide some sources for additional information. There are still more sources included in my earlier book, *Chemical Exposure and Disease: Diagnostic and Investigative Techniques,* but for the present book, I have tried to give a variety of sources, so this is not an exhaustive list. To other activist writers and worthy organizations whose work is not included, I apologize. I urge readers to pursue their own paths to learning and awareness. These citations cover cancer in general, breast cancer specifically, nuclear and x-ray radiation, chemical toxicity, pesticides, drugs, and some of the underlying political and economic pressures that contribute to cancer. I have included some references on ethics and social thought. Some of the citations cover several points of view in the same volume. When a book is published by a small press, the address and price are supplied.

I have included as well, names and address of breast cancer activist and environmental organizations in the United States and Canada that provide information, education, and support.

RADIATION-INDUCED CANCER

Deadly Deceit: Low-Level Radiation, High-Level Cover-Up
Jay M. Gould and Benjamin A. Goldman
Four Walls, Eight Windows Press. PO Box 548, Village Station, NY
1991 ($10.95)

> An investigation of governmental and industry records of radiation releases
> and the link to cancer, birth defects, and immunological failure. The maps of
> nuclear reactor sites provide fallout patterns from each of the facilities, and
> the well-thought-out graphs support the text data.

**Preventing Breast Cancer: The Story of a Major, Proven, Preventable Cause of this
      Disease.**
John W. Gofman, M.D., Ph.D.
Committee for Nuclear Responsibility, Inc., PO Box 412993, San Francisco, CA
94142
Second Edition: 1996 ($17.00)

> An easy-to-read and scholarly compendium of findings linking past use of x-ray
> radiation in causing breast cancer. These practices include x-ray treatment of
> tonsils, thymus radiation of children, for shoe-fitting, x-rays for skin disease, and
> past and current mammography. It emphasizes there is no level of exposure
> below which this is no risk.

The Enemy Within: The High Cost of Living Near Nuclear Reactors
Jay Gould
Four Walls, Eight Windows Press
PO Box 548, Village Station, NY
1996 ($14.95)

> The author is the director of the baby teeth study to determine environmental
> radioactive strontium levels.

Multiple Exposure: Chronicles of the Radiation Age
Catherine Caufield
University of Chicago Press, Chicago, IL
1989

> The industrial-governmental complex at work in contamination from nuclear
> weapons and power development.

X-Rays: Health Effects of Common Exams
John W. Gofman, M.D., Ph.D., and Egan O'Connor
Sierra Club Books, San Francisco, CA
1985

> A practical guide that sorts the high-risk medical and dental x-rays from the
> low-risk ones, with easy-to-use tables by age and sex. This is a useful reference
> for patients, parents, physicians, and dentists.

Radiation and Human Health: A comprehensive investigation of the evidence relating low-level radiation to cancer and other diseases
John W. Gofman, M.D., Ph.D.
Sierra Club Books, San Francisco, CA, 908 pages
1981

> A treasure-house of information and supporting data that long ago should have been used to stop nuclear development, and that can be used today. Dr. Gofman is eminently qualified on the issues of nuclear radiation and human health. He is both a physician and a doctor of nuclear/physical chemistry.

Radioactive Heaven and Earth: The Health and Environmental Effects of Nuclear Weapons Testing In, On, and Above the Earth.
International Physicians for the Prevention of Nuclear War (IPPNW)
Apex Press, Council on International and Public Affairs
777 United Nations Plaza, New York, NY 10017
1991

> This small paperback documents adverse effects of global weapons testing with emphasis on cancer of various organs.

Refuge: An Unnatural History of Family and Place
Terry Tempest Williams
Vintage Books, Division of Random House, Inc.
New York ($12.00)
1991

> This stunning book, written with love and grace, is an account of the beauty of the earth, transformed by the nuclear test legacy. The message is impossible to ignore.

Nuclear Information and Resource Service (NIRS)
1424 16th Street, N.W., Suite 404
Washington, D.C. 20036
202-328-0002
e-mail: nirsnet@igc.org
website: www.nirs.org

> NIRS was founded in 1978 by grassroots activists committed to a nonnuclear energy policy. The organization provides information and grassroots networking.

Abolition 2000
Nuclear Age Peace Foundation
1187 Coast Village Road, #123, Santa Barbara, CA 93108
805-965-3443
e-mail:wagingpeace@napf.org

Chernobyl—Environmental, Health and Human Rights Implications
Permanent People's Tribunal,

International Medical Commission on Chernobyl (IMCC)
IMCC, 710-264 Queens Quay, West
Toronto, Ontario M5J 1B5, Canada
e-mail:103062.1200@compuserve.com
and
Global Educational Associates
475 Riverside Drive, Suite 1848
New York, NY 10115
212-870-3290

> This is a stunning transcription of testimony by scientists, victims, and those who worked at the site after the Chernobyl catastrophe. It is "undiluted" and a must for anyone who wants to know the true consequences of exposure to nuclear radiation.

Breast Cancer and Radioactive Strontium in Baby Teeth
Radiation and Public Health Project
PO Box 60, Unionville, NY 10988
1-800-582-3716

> When you call this number, you will be given information on where and how to send children's teeth for assays of radioactive strontium (Sr 90). The results will be coded by zip codes to determine if there is a correlation between Sr-90 levels, breast and other cancers.

The Final Epidemic
Ruth Adams and Susan Cullen, Editors
Education Foundation for Nuclear Science, Inc.
1020 East 58th Street, Chicago, IL 60637
(Distributed by the University of Chicago Press)
1981

> A compendium of essays by leading physicians and scientists, showing the effects of nuclear war and steps we must take to stop the arms race.

ENDOCRINE DISRUPTION/CANCER AND REPRODUCTIVE FAILURE

Our Stolen Future
Theo Colborn, Ph.D., Dianne Dumanoski, and John Peterson Myers, Ph.D
Dutton, Penguin Books
USA, Canada, England, Australia, New Zealand
1996

> This book traces the spread of chemicals that interfere with reproduction at very low levels, and documents genital and reproductive abnormalities in wild animals, and alterations in brain function. The implications for future survival of humans and wildlife is profound.

Chemically-Induced Alterations in Sexual and Functional Development: The Wildlife/Human Connection.
Theo Colborn and Coralie Clement, Editors
Princeton Scientific Publishing Co., Inc. Princeton, NJ
1992

> A collection of papers given at a workshop in 1991. It documents abnormalities in animals as a result of chemicals interfering with endocrine function, and provided background for the above publication.

Generations At Risk
Greater Boston PSR
1996
617-497-7440
e-mail: psrmabo@igc.org

> While emphasizing Massachusetts, this 150-page publication shows how environmental toxins may affect reproductive health.

Women and the Crisis in Sex Hormones
Barbara Seaman and Gideon Seaman
Bantam books, New York, NY, Toronto, London, and Sydney
1977

> A best seller, available in paperback, reveals what everyone should know who has taken, or is thinking of taking, hormones.

BRAIN DAMAGE

Chemical Brain Injury
Kaye H. Kilburn, MD
1998
John Wiley and Sons, Publisher, New York, NY
1-800-225-5945

> A clinician's study of patients exposed to chemicals that altered forever their ability to think and function. Many communities with high cancer rates also find neurological dysfunction as well. Many chemicals are both neurotoxic and carcinogenic.

POLITICS AND ECONOMICS OF DISEASE

Inconclusive By Design: Waste Fraud and Abuse in Federal Environmental Health Research
Environmental Health Network and the National Toxics Campaign
PO Box 16267, Chesapeake, VA 23328-6267
1992 ($15.00)

This 55-page volume is a must for anyone contemplating participation in a university or governmental "study" of a community. Beware the pitfalls!

Contaminated Communities: The Social and Psychological Impacts of Residential Toxic Exposure
Michael R. Edelstein

Westview Press, Boulder, CO, and London, England

1988

Chemical contamination, the varying definition of "risk," the inability/refusal of governmental help, and how communities have and have not achieved a safe environment.

Dying from Dioxin
Lois Marie Gibbs

South End Press

116 Saint Botolph Street, Boston, MA 02115

1995

361 pages, $20.00

Understandable information on the chemistry, biology, and politics of dioxin contamination, where it comes from, and how to mobilize to counteract this threat to health and the environment.

Toxic Deception: How the Chemical Industry Manipulated Science, Bends the Law, and Endangers Your Health
Dan Fagan and Marianne Lavelle

Birch Lane Press, 120 Enterprise Ave., Seacaucus, NJ 07094

Canadian Manda Group, One Atlantic Ave. Suite 105, Toronto M6K 3E7 Canada

1996

This volume, written with support form the Center For Public Integrity, backs up its title with names, associations, and follows the money trial linking pollution and politics.

Toxic Sludge is Good for You—Lies, Damn Lies, and the Public Relations Industry
John Stauber and Sheldon Rampton

Common Courage Press, Monroe, ME

1995

Is just what the title says. Needed to understand where so much "information" comes from and how to assess its the accuracy and/or truth.

When Corporations Rule the World
David C. Korten

Kumarian Press, 14 Oakwood Ave., W. Hartford, CT 06119-2127

1995 ($19.95)

Documentation of the devastating consequences of economic globalization by transnational corporations and compliant governments, where workers, customers, services, and products have become secondary to monetary profit.

Corporate Crime and Violence: Big Business and the Abuse of the Public Trust
Russell Mokhiber

Sierra Club Books, San Francisco, CA

1988 ($16.00)

> Quoting from the book cover: "The thing for you to do is buy this book and read all these case histories and all his remedies. That should motivate you to corner your senators and congressmen and threaten to tie them down and force feed them coal dust, bad baby formula, Oraflex and asbestos, if they don't agree to help us out. Now."

Trading Freedom—How Free Trade Affects Our Lives, Work, and Environment
J. Cavanagh, J. Gershman, K. Baker, G. Helmke, Editors

Institute for Food Development Policy

145 Ninth Street, San Francisco, CA 94103

1992 ($10.00)

> This slim book focuses on NAFTA, the North American Free Trade Agreement, and how it affects workers, agriculture, human rights, immigration, agriculture, and the threat of control by transnational corporations. The book outlines alternative paths for a sustainable environment, while providing social justice, democracy, and equality.

A Civil Action
Jonathan Harr

Random House, New York, NY

1995

> The true story of residents of Woburn, MA, who developed cancer as a result of exposure to chemicals, and their subsequent, very difficult, legal battles. It was voted "Best Book of the Year" by Entertainment Weekly.

Love Canal—My Story
Lois Gibbs

State University of New York Press

Albany, NY

1982

> This book details the struggles of the residents of Love Canal against corporate and governmental interests. It is available from the Center for Health, Environment and Justice, PO Box 6806, Falls Church, VA 22040

PESTICIDES AND ILLNESSES

Silent Spring
Rachel Carson

Houghton Mifflin, New York (original publisher)

1962

This book must be read again and again. Written 35 years ago, it is still true. If anything, it documents how much we know of the adverse effects of chemical exposure, and how little we have accomplished in prevention.

A Canary's Tale
Jacob Berkson

PO Box 2041, Hagerstown, MD 21742-2041

1996 ($19.95)

The author, poisoned in his own home by a pesticide, traces the link between "low-level" exposure to chemicals and adverse effects, including cancer, asthma, multiple chemical sensitivity (MCS). The last, MCS patients, are like the canary in the coal mine, warning that the environment is polluted, and sounding a call for action.

Our Children's Toxic Legacy—How Science and Law Fail to Protect Us from Pesticides
John Wargo, M. D.

Yale University of Press, New Haven, CT, and London

1996

An exceptional book tracing the history of pesticides, and the link between pesticides and cancer, neurological effects, and environmental contamination.

The Pesticide Conspiracy
Robert Van den Bosch

Doubleday, Garden City, NY

1978

This book may be out of print, but is well worth getting from a library. Written two decades ago, it warned of what was to follow if pesticide use was not curbed. Unfortunately, Van den Bosch's findings have come true.

Diet for a Poisoned Planet
David Steinman

Harmony Books/Crown Publishers, Inc., New York, NY

1990

This is an easy book to read. Using official governmental data from EPA and FDA sources, the author documents pesticide and hormone contamination of food, and rates foods safe and unsafe to eat. Available in paperback.

Designer Poisons: How to Protect your Health and Home from Toxic Pesticides
Marion Moses, M.D.

Pesticide Education Center

PO Box 420870, San Francisco, CA 94142-0870

1995 ($19.95)

A guide to how to reduce our risk of cancer and other diseases by reducing exposure to pesticides, and by providing alternative solutions to these problems.

OVEREXPOSED: Organophosphate Insecticides in Children's Food
Richard Wiles, Kert Davies, and Christopher Campbell
Environmental Working Group
1718 Connecticut Avenue, N.W., Suite 600, Washington, D.C., 20009
1998 ($20.00)

> A careful analysis of food-pesticide data that concludes that every day
> more than one million children age 5 and under eat an unsafe diet of
> organophosphate pesticides, having the potential to cause long-term
> damage to the brain and nervous system.

ETHICS AND SOCIAL THOUGHT

Downsize This!
Michael Moore
Crown Publishers, Inc.
New York, NY 10022
1996

> An irreverent and clear look at corporations, economics politicians, unemploy-
> ment, and current culture, presented with irony and humor. This book, and his
> previous book and film of the same name, *Roger and Me,* are a must. So too is
> his film *The Big One.* Perhaps the answer to much of our cancer and environ-
> mental degradation could be remedied by using these books and films as texts
> in our schools.

Global Bioethics
Van Renssalaer Potter
Michigan State University Press, East Lansing, MI
1988

> Dr. Potter builds on the legacy of Aldo Leopold. He combines science and
> humanistic knowledge to set priorities for acceptable survival, stressing ethics
> and morality. Small paperback book, filled with thought.

Ideas and Opinions
Albert Einstein
Wings Books, Random House, New York, NY
1954

> Essays by the master himself, covering atomic energy, government, politics,
> economics, war, education, ethics, etc. It is a refreshing view of a profound
> thinker.

The Closing Circle—Nature, Man and Technology
Barry Commoner
Bantam Books, New York, NY
1971

What concerned Dr. Commoner appears not to have improved. His book is worth reading again, if we are to save ourselves and our only world.

The Ages of Gaia—A Biography of Our Living Earth
James Lovelock

W. W. Norton, New York, NY

1988

> A view of the earth as a single, living organism with each individual component, dependent upon others for life and sustenance. We would be wise to understand the consequences of pollution and imbalances created by loss of species, and changes in the atmosphere and in the seas.

The Lives of a Cell
Lewis Thomas

Bantam Books, New York, NY

1974

> A thoughtful consideration of the uniqueness of life. Dr. Lewis explores cancer, disease, the interdependency of all life: what we take so for granted.

HEALTH, ADVOCACY, AND INFORMATION ORGANIZATIONS

American Environmental Health Foundation
8345 Walnut Hill Lane, Suite 225, Dallas, TX 75231-44262

214-361-9515

FAX 691-8432

> Physicians and allied health workers, trained to recognize environmentally related diseases, guide the patient to avoid exposure, and provide treatment regimes to decrease intrinsic toxic chemical load.

Association of Birth Defects Children (ABDC)
900 Woodcock Road, Suite 225, Orlando, FL 32803

407-245-7035

800-313-2232

> This organization maintains a registry on children with birth defects, and collects such information as in utero exposures as pesticides, drugs, silicone implants, service in the Gulf War etc.

Breast Cancer Action
55 New Montgomery Street, #624, San Francisco, CA 94105

415-243-9301

FAX 243-3996

e-mail: bcaction@hooked.net

> The aim of this group is "to make breast cancer a national priority through education and advocacy; to promote and refocus research into the causes, prevention, treatment and cure of breast cancer, and to empower women and men to participate fully in decisions relating to breast cancer."

Cancer Awareness Coalition
PO Box 533, New Paltz, NY 12561

> A very effective grassroots organization, dedicated to exposing sources of chemical pollution and promoting prevention in their area. New Paltz is located in the lower Hudson River Valley amid a fruit-growing region and an area of high breast cancer incidence.

CATS (Californians for Alternatives to Toxics)
PO Box 1195, Arcata, CA 95518

707-822-8497

e-mail:cats@igc.org

webpage: www.mapcruzin.com/cats

> The group has low-cost publications concerning pesticide use on public lands, roadsides, and agriculture, as well as forest management and other resources.

Center for Community Action and Environmental Justice
P.O. Box 33124, Riverside, CA 92519

909-360-8451

> Publications include: Women, Cancer and Environment, Asian/Pacific Islander Environmental Justice, Communities at Risk Network and Rural Communities Project, all available for a nominal sum.

Center for Health, Environment and Justice
(Previously Citizens Clearinghouse for Hazardous Waste)
PO Box 6806, Falls Church, VA 22040

703-237-2249

> This was the organization organized by Lois Gibbs in response to the Love Canal contamination. Since then, it has become a nationwide source for communities and citizens concerned about contamination. CHEJ provides information and organizational strategies.

Complementary & Alternative Medicine at the NIH
Office of Alternative Medicine

National Institutes of Health

Building 31, 5B-38, Bethesda, MD 20892

888-644-6226

website:altmed.od.nih.gov

> The Office of Alternative Medicine identifies and evaluates unconventional health care practices; conducts research and training on these practices and disseminates information.

Environmental Defense Fund
1616 P Street, N.W., Washington, D.C. 20036

202- 387-3500

website:www.scorecard.org

> An important service is the new internet site where any person can access the chemical Scorecard by corporation, zip code, map, health effects, chemicals, and regulatory controls. A true public service. This is an established organization supporting research and publication of health and environmental issues.

Environmental Health Perspectives

National Institute of Environmental Health Sciences (NIEHS)

PO Box 12233, Research Triangle Park, NC 27709-2233

> NIEHS is a division of the Public Health Service and the National Institutes of Health. For a governmental agency, this is an uncommon publication of important articles on the link between environmental contamination and illness.

Food and Water Journal

RR 1, Box 68D, Walden , VT 05873 ($25.00 per year)

802-563-3300

800-EAT-SAFE

> A well-written, monthly publication that looks at such topics at bovine growth hormone, food radiation, pesticides, and various laws that support their use.

Green Guide

A publication of Mothers and Others

40 W. 20th Street, New York, NY 10011-4211

888-ECO-INFO

> Monthly publication on chemical and radiation exposure issues of importance to mothers, and others, and their children.

Jeremiah Project

Shepherd of the Hills Presbyterian Church

222 Soft Wind, Canyon Lake, TX 78133

> An interdenominational ministry for people who are chemically sensitive and/or have been chemically injured. It works toward "education of others about the harm that overuse of chemicals has caused all of creation, including the human species." Provides information about chemicals and reviews books.

League of Conservation Voters

1707 L Street, N.W., Suite 750, Washington, D.C. 20036

202-785-8683

website: http://www.lcv.org

> This group keeps track of environmental issues before Congress. In their most recent tally (available on their website), 46 percent of U.S. Congress members voted pro-environment for only one of 16 environmental votes that came before the Congress.

National Women's Health Network

514 Tenth Street, N.W. #400, Washington, D. C. 20004

202-628-7814

> This group issues collections of very useful publications and the sources, names, and addresses of others working on specific issues. Booklets on Breast Cancer, sold for a reasonable fee of $6.00 for members and $8.00 for nonmembers include the following subjects:
>
> Detection/ Diagnosis
>
> Diethylstilbestrol (DES)

Environmental Causes
Implants (Saline)
Menopause: Alternative Therapies
Prevention/ Risk Factors
Tamoxifen: "Prevention Trials"
Treatment/ Recovery
　and more

Pennsylvania Breast Cancer Coalition

Doneckers Complex

55 New Street, Suite 5, Ephrata, PA 17522

717-738-9567

800-475-9880

Active advocacy and support group, with local chapters throughout the state. It originated the photo display of women with breast cancer from every county in the state.

Physicians for Social Responsibility

1101 Fourteenth Street, N.W., Suite 700, Washington, D.C. 20005

202-898-0150

webpage:www.psr.org

Originally organized to achieve the end of nuclear arms, the organization is involved in an international effort to phase out 12 toxins. These are DDT; the related pesticides aldrin, dieldrin, endrin, chlordane, and heptachlor; the pesticides hexachlorobenzene, mirex, and toxaphene; and the pollutants dioxins and furans. While there has been progress in the U.S., Canada, and the U. K., both China and India are far from banning these persistent chemicals.

Rachel Carson Council

8940 Jones Mill Road, Chevy Chase, MD 20815

301-652-1877

e-mail:rccouncil@aol.com

Named after Ms. Carson, who died of breast cancer, the organization provides information on pesticides (toxicology on existing chemicals and alternatives). It has excellent publications, including one on breast cancer.

Rachel's Environment and Health Weekly

Environmental Research Foundation

105 Eastern Avenue - Suite 101, Annapolis, MD 21403-3300

405-263-1584

FAX 263-8944

e-mail: erf@rachel.clark.net

An extraordinary publication covering a wide range of issues concerning public health: toxic chemicals, environmental information; legal, ethical, and political aspects.

Toxinformer
Environmental Health Coalition
1717 Kettner Blvd., Suite 100, San Diego, CA 92101-2532
619-235-0281
e-mail:ehcoalition@igc.apc.org
webpage:www.environmentalhealth.org

> The group is dedicated to the prevention and cleanup of toxic pollution; promotes environmental justice; monitors government and industry actions that cause pollution; and educates communities about toxic hazards and toxics use reduction. The news publication is printed in English and Spanish.

Virginia Breast Cancer Foundation
PO Box 17884, Richmond, VA 23226
1-800-345-VBCF

> An active advocacy and support group, that issues legislative alerts in the interests of breast cancer patients.

Women's Community Cancer Project
The Women's Center
46 Pleasant Street, Cambridge, MA 02139
617-354-9888

> This is a grassroots volunteer organization committed to facilitating change in the medical, social, and political approaches to cancer, particularly as they affect women. One of their efforts includes "Breast Cancer and the Environment: MAKE THE CONNECTION"

WEDO—Women's Environment and Development Organization
355 Lexington, Avenue, 3rd Floor, New York, NY 10017-6603
212-973-0325
FAX 973-0335
e-mailwedo@igc.apc.org
webpage: http://www.wedo.org

> Former U.S. House of Representative member Bella S. Abzug was co-chair of this organization. This group makes the connection between contamination of the environment and the increasing incidence of breast cancer. Their aim is for meaningful research into prevention of illness.WEDO is an accredited non-governmental organization with consultative status at the United Nations, thus in a position to push for women's health policy worldwide.

CANADIAN ADVOCACY ORGANIZATIONS

Canadian Breast Cancer Network
102-207 Rue Bank Street, Ottawa, Ontario K2P 2N2, Canada
613-788-3311
FAX 233-1056

> This group has given emphasis on environmental chemical and breast cancer.

First Nations' Breast Cancer Society
Woman's Hospital and Health Center
4500 Oak Street, Room D-311
Vancouver, British Columbia V6H 3N1, Canada
604-875-3677
FAX 875-2445

> This nonprofit organization group addresses the cancer problems of native Canadians.

World Conference on Breast Cancer
841 Princess Street, Kingston, Ontario, K7L 1G7, Canada
613-549-1118
FAX 549-1146

> This group of volunteers organized the meeting of advocates from 60 countries to establish a GLOBAL ACTION PLAN FOR BREAST CANCER.

Women's Network on Health
736 Bathurst Street, Toronto, Ontario M5S 2R4, Canada
416-516-2600

> The video *Exposure—Environmental Links to Breast Cancer,* and the companion booklet Taking Action for a Health Future are invaluable guides to the link between pollution and breast cancer. The organization has a very useful list of printed, film, video and radio sources as well. There are resources listed for women in Canada, Asia, Europe, South America, the Caribbean, and globally.

INDEX

The letter *f* after a number indicates that a figure is on the page.